PROFESSIONAL DOMINANCE

PROFESSIONAL DOMINANCE

The Social Structure of Medical Care

Eliot Freidson

Routledge
Taylor & Francis Group
LONDON AND NEW YORK

First published 1970 by Transaction Publishers

Published 2017 by Routledge
2 Park Square, Milton Park, Abingdon, Oxon OX14 4RN
711 Third Avenue, New York, NY 10017, USA

First issued in hardback 2017

Routledge is an imprint of the Taylor & Francis Group, an informa business

Library of Congress Catalog Number: 2006045680

Library of Congress Cataloging-in-Publication Data

Freidson, Eliot, 1923-2005.
Professional dominance: the social structure of medical care / Eliot Freidson.—lst pbk. ed.
p. cm.
Includes bibliographical references.
ISBN 0-202-30855-3 (pbk. : alk. paper)
1. Social medicine. 2. Medical care—United States. I. Title.

RA418F74 2006
362.10973-dc22 2006045680

ISBN 13: 978-1-138-53086-7 (hbk)
ISBN 13: 978-0-202-30855-5 (pbk)

for Judy

Contents

FOREWORD, ix
INTRODUCTION: Substantive Issues in Medical Sociology, 1

Part 1. A Sociological Approach to Medical Care

1. The Present State of Medical Sociology, 41
2. A Structural Approach to Medical Care, 59

Part 2. The Position of the Profession in the Medical Care Structure

3. The Profession—An Overview, 81
4. The Structural Solution to the Problem of Professional Authority, 105
5. Professional Dominance and the Ordering of Health Services, 127

Part 3. Problems of Organizing Medical Care

6. Organizing Hospital Care, 167
7. Organizing Ambulatory Medical Care, 187
8. Professional Dominance and the Reorganization of Medical Care, 209

INDEX, 239

Foreword

In the United States today we are confronted by a number of serious social problems, not the least of which concern the character of our basic human services. In each of the broad public domains of welfare, education, law, and health there are crises of public confidence. Each in its own way is failing to accomplish its essential mission of alleviating material deprivation, instructing the young, controlling and righting criminal and civil wrongs, and healing the sick. The poor, the student, the offender and the victim, the sick —all have in some way protested the failure of the institutions responsible for them. And these protests occur at a time when the human services are absorbing an increasingly massive amount of money and manpower.

Awareness of that crisis intensified in the 1960s, and increasing energy has been invested in research designed to determine what can be done. Each of the human services has long had its own research tradition, but during the sixties each has also made a concerted effort to mobilize and use the skills of such comparatively new disciplines as sociology. Owing to these new demands, sociology itself has grown. The hitherto obscure specialties of the sociology of law and medicine and the established specialties of criminology and educational sociology have taken on new vigor. In applying themselves to the task of studying the human services, however, these segments of sociology have had to choose between two different strategies.

The most common approach of sociology to practical affairs has been to make its technical skills of data collection and its special descriptive concepts available to the institutions and occupations of the human services. Such an approach has supplemented and deepened the research of those services and has provided them with more information about themselves and their tasks than they had before. It is certainly important and useful, but by its very nature it takes as given the underlying assumptions as well as the basic structure of the services it studies. If these underlying assumptions happen to be incorrect, research based on them cannot have more than limited, short-run value. Similarly, if the basic structure of those services is responsible for significant failings, merely studying and changing what goes on within the structure cannot lead to more than superficial amelioration.

A second approach is the one I shall adopt in this book. Rather than dealing with the details of the human services for their own sake—and this lack of detail is a characteristic limitation of the second approach—I shall instead attempt to stand outside the system in order to delineate one of its critical assumptions and a strategic feature of its basic structure. In doing so, I shall deal with the concept of profession, for as I shall try to show, the concept rests on assumptions about how services to laymen should be controlled and is realized by a special kind of social structure that organizes the presentation of those services. The consequences for the operation of the system of services are, I shall argue, pervasive and profound. Indeed, in the case of health, which is the most professionalized of all the human services, the power of the concept is such that it has even influenced the way medical sociologists have studied it.

In the concrete case of health services, how is the concept of profession manifested? First, it may be noted that in matters of health the opinions of laymen are very likely to be subordinated to the opinions of professional experts. This subordination is based on the assumption that a professional has such special esoteric knowledge and humanitarian intent that he and he alone should be allowed to decide what is good for the layman. This assumption forms the ideological foundation of health and other highly professionalized human services. On this foundation is built a form of organization much different from that found in the management of ordinary commercial services and industrial enterprises. Health services are organized around professional authority, and their basic structure is constituted by the dominance of a single profession over a variety of other, subordinate occupations. I shall argue that professional dominance is the analytical key to the present inadequacy of the health services. And while I shall restrict details almost entirely to the field of health, my intent is to suggest that there are serious deficiencies in the nature of professionalism in general and that it can be shown to be responsible for problems in the other human services as well.

Some of the material in this book has been published elsewhere in an earlier form. I wish to acknowledge with gratitude the permission of the publishers to use sections of my work from the following publications: *Institutions and the Person*, eds. Howard S. Becker, Blanche Geer, David Riesman, and Robert S. Weiss (Chicago: Aldine Publishing Company, 1968), copyright © 1968 by Howard

S. Becker, Blanche Geer, David Riesman, and Robert S. Weiss; a volume edited by Mark Lefton and William R. Rosengren to be published in 1970 by Charles E. Merrill Publishing Co.; *Social Problems*, 14 (Spring 1967), 493–500, copyright 1967 by the Society for the Study of Social Problems; *Current Sociology*, 10–11 (1961–1962), 123–192, copyright 1963 by Basil Blackwell & Matt Ltd.; and *International Encyclopedia of Social Sciences*, ed. David L. Sills (New York: Macmillan, 1968), vol. 10, pp. 105–113, copyright © 1968 by Crowell Collier and Macmillan, Inc.

Finally, I should like to acknowledge with gratitude the helpful comments of Judith Lorber, George A. Silver, and Harold Wise.

Introduction: Substantive Issues in Medical Sociology

In the rather short time it has been in existence as a recognizable specialty, medical sociology has sprawled across a vast array of substantive areas without any obvious rationale for its coverage, and medical sociologists' approaches to its study have been so varied as to defy integration.[1] Indeed, while two recent books have addressed themselves to the field, both are extremely selective, omitting much of the substantive field. One limits itself largely to social aspects of disease and the social processes leading to the adoption of the sick role,[2] and the other limits itself to an analysis of the medical profession.[3] The present book is also limited to but a portion of the material included in the field. In fact, it will limit itself to a rather narrow segment of the field—specifically, that segment bearing on the way in which health services are presented to the consumer in the United States. But narrow or not, I shall argue that the organization of health services has consequences of great importance in many other areas. I shall argue, furthermore, that a truly sophisticated and useful analysis of a concrete topic such as the organization of health services requires the use of rather general and abstract sociological concepts. Much of my exposition will in fact be devoted to elaborating these concepts rather than to describing the complex and rapidly changing data connected with the delivery of medical care in this or any other industrialized society. In elaborating these concepts I hope to contribute both to the practical problem of formulating concrete social policies for the health services and to the theoretical problem of creating a genuine sociology of medicine.

To place this contribution in the context of the entire field of medical sociology, however, it seems appropriate to describe the whole sprawling breadth of that field. This I shall attempt to do now, following the description by a discussion of the relation of this book to the field. Throughout, I shall attempt to deal with the substantive as well as the conceptual issues of the field. My presentation will begin with a discussion of the bearing of the idea of disease on the concepts of social control and deviance, which will pose a challenge to studies in the tradition of the sociology of knowledge. After a brief review of the problem of explanation raised by studies of the distribution of disease, extended attention will be paid to the relevance of the concept of social role to the behavior of people who are sick and those whom they consult. Discussion of the role of the healing consultant will lead to consideration of the concept of profession and such contingent questions as recruitment, the nature of professional training, practice, and interprofessional relations. This will be followed by a consideration of the hospital and like institutions in the context provided by the concept of bureaucratic organization, and, finally, a very brief consideration of health affairs and health institutions within the framework of the community. Given that context, I shall then attempt to specify the place of the study of medical care in the field of medical sociology.

The Concept of Disease

The most general question sociology may ask about medicine concerns the knowledge and ideas that surround it. A very large body of historical materials as well as a somewhat more scattered body of ethnographic reporting allows any number of questions to be investigated in considerable detail.[4] The most conventional investigations, which historians have most often performed, are addressed to the state of scientific medical knowledge in a particular historical period, the biographies of medical men, and the circumstances surrounding a particular scientific discovery. But only a handful of historians[5] has been seriously concerned with such specifically sociological questions as the determination of medical theories by prevailing religious or political philosophies of the time, the relation of the class system to the medical division of labor, the development of modern professionalism, and even the characteristic social contingencies of medical practice. It is not as if data are lacking for such analyses, for as the Wellcome Library's periodical publication indicates, there is an enormous number of primary and secondary materials available.[6] One may hope that sociologists, if not historians, may make more use of such material in the future.

Apart from historical analysis there is the somewhat different problem involving the definition of disease as such. In practice the notion of disease is at once an objective and an evaluative or moral concept.[7] It contains not only an at least substantively rational attempt at explanation of cause and specification of cure but also, if only implicitly, an indication of responsibility for the condition. Quite obviously, if an undesirable ailment is believed to be divine punishment for sinful behavior, its occurrence has different social consequences than when it is believed to be the result of malicious human witchcraft, willful perversity, or impersonal, material forces over which no one has control. Many kinds of human complaints that we now call diseases have at one time or another been considered to be of such varied causes.

It seems fairly hopeless for the sociologist to work with the idea that there are objective disease states even though there is no doubt they exist. It is true that there are some conditions, like a distinctly broken leg, that all men everywhere would agree on. But it is also true that there are many other conditions of which we were not aware until recently, of which other people are not now aware, and of which we are not yet aware. Furthermore, "natural" states recognized everywhere to exist may or may not be treated as disease; pregnancy, for example, can be perceived as a natural and normal state or as an illness to be rejected;[8] drug habituation can be viewed as a disease or as a crime.[9] These confusions in definition occur in the idea of disease only if we insist on the objectivity of the designation. For the sociologist it is quite beside the point whether or not the designation of disease is objective, for the designation, right or wrong, real or imaginary, has social consequences in any case. Because the task of determining the "real" existence and cause of disease is left for the physician, the sociologist can study the social consequences of *imputing* disease and what kind of social concept disease is.

Talcott Parsons has discussed disease as one type of deviance requiring control by society.[10] As a social concept, the imputation of disease in modern society labels particular kinds of undesired or unexpected behavior as due to natural causes for whose operation the deviant may not be held responsible and which are amenable to control by the uses of natural techniques of therapy. The behavior in question may or may not "really" be disease as scientific medicine might define it, and, in one or another historical time or place, may be defined as deviance of quite another class or may not even be recognized as deviance at all. The sociologist, then, may treat disease as a type of social deviance that has specific social consequences. Indeed, he may examine the use of the concept of disease in modern times as a social movement and as a problem in the sociology of knowledge.

Disease as Ideology

Modern times are witness to the inclusion of more behavior under the concept of disease than ever before. Just as the simple Newtonian world is being displaced by the considerably more diffuse world of modern physics, so is the simple world of Pasteur being displaced by one in which direct causal relationship between "germ" and disease is being questioned and in which notions like stress come to play mediating if not causal roles. The idea of stress, however, brings to the fore the complicated and obscure psychological and social variables that heretofore could be treated by the diagnostician as if they did not exist. Thus the naturalistic stance of medicine has moved from the biological into the psychological and social realm, coming to consider the latter as part of the "disease" addressed and legitimized by the former.

Perhaps more important than the idea of stress was the development of a medical orientation to mental disorder, much of which in medical knowledge is only obscurely connected with biophysical processes. The idea that personal and social inadequacy has rationally determinable origins amenable to purposive change or cure was, of course, not created by Freud, but it may be said that not until his work and that of his followers has its acceptance become almost a matter of orthodoxy. The growing acceptance of that idea has encouraged the inclusion of a tremendous number of social and psychological phenomena under the category of disease, phenomena which hitherto had been considered largely in moral, legal, or other terms. Expansion of the category of supposedly morally neutral, scientifically detached "disease" does not seem to have been guided solely by scientific evidence. It seems closely related to the secular, liberal, humanitarian ideology, as a number of analysts have suggested.[11]

This view of man and his ills has several important characteristics. First of all, in ascribing natural disease to many areas of human behavior which hitherto were not so regarded, it designates as pathological and amenable to scientific treatment what once was held to be a consequence of responsible personal choice or of an irrevocable state of sin or genetic inferiority. Moral arguments for social reform become displaced by "scientific" arguments. Second, it creates a rhetoric by which behavior the actor believes to be serious and responsible, even if deviant, is reduced to a mere symptom of disease for which he is not truly responsible. For example, those who hold extreme political beliefs, whether radical or ultra-conservative, have been called sick because of their beliefs, thus denying the validity of debating those beliefs on their own merits. Another result, however, is not to punish those whose behavior is deviant, but to treat them, a result that threatens the traditional functions of the courts.

Aside from the extreme cases of generally acknowledged lunacy and unpremeditated crimes of passion, for which the argument of irresponsibility holds sway, the courts have regarded most adult behavior to be deliberate and calculating, men making choices for which they may be held responsible and punished. Laws, courts, and prisons have been predicated upon such an assumption. But the new view of man has tended to encourage the assumption that some kinds of "disease," whether of society or the individual or his immediate environment, cause crime, and that therefore the criminal should not be punished but treated. Since the courts have had the historic function of determining and assigning responsibility and retribution, one may easily understand why in one study lawyers were found to be less "enlightened" about mental illness than their peers in other occupations; their very ideology, part of their professional stance, specifies responsibility where lack of responsibility is now being claimed.[12] The resistance of people committed to an ethic of responsibility is strengthened by the inadequacy of much of the evidence supporting this view of man, but it is weakened, one might suspect, by the humanitarian quality of its sentimental appeal.

If there is patent evidence that those who are responsible for extending the concept of natural disease to cover more and more types of social deviance are members of the liberal bourgeoisie, there is considerably less evidence about the identity of those who resist the extension. One very interesting discussion for the United States links nonhumanitarian attitudes toward crime and mental illness with the Puritan ideology.[13] An empirical study of "nonhumanism" in hospital attendants finds it correlated with "authoritarianism,"[14] which itself seems to be a working-class trait. A study of negative attitudes toward medicine as such refers to the "Protestant ethic."[15] Finally, a study of leaders of local groups opposed to the fluoridation of drinking water suggested that their antipathy was part of a more general sense of alienation from the new scientific society.[16] There is also evidence that the poorly educated are less likely than the well educated to consider their physical and mental "problems" to be illnesses or to be serious enough to require professional medical attention.[17]

Social Elements in the Distribution and Etiology of Illness

It has been suggested that the proper interest of the physician lies in the study of what he believes to be disease, while that of the sociologist lies in the study of the behavior surrounding scientifically diagnosed disease and imputed disease. The sociologist, however, can make a contribution to the medical task by indicating some of the social correlates of disease and thereby suggesting possible elements in its etiology.

One question that has received a great deal of attention from medical people has been the distribution of illness, for knowledge of its distribution can supply hints of cause.[18] A variety of social variables has been found of significance in ordering the distribution of disease. Some illness is rare outside particular occupations because particular kinds of work bring the worker into contact with causative agents not met by others in the normal course of their lives.[19] "Black lung disease" among miners and cancer of the scrotum among chimney sweeps are obvious cases. Other illnesses are said to occur most frequently among particular ethnic and racial groups—whether the significant variable lies in diet or other peculiar customs, in general standard of living, or in genetics varies from one illness and one group to another. Still other illnesses occur most characteristically among particular economic groups, some a result of the filth of poverty and others, like paralytic poliomyelitis, a result of the asepsis of wealth.

While it establishes connections, the epidemiological method does not by itself establish cause. In some instances there is tantalizing ambiguity in the problem of distinguishing cause from effect. In the case of chronic illness in the United States, where no national health scheme makes care available to everyone irrespective of income, it is not clear whether the environment surrounding a low socioeconomic position is the cause or the effect of chronic illness. A similar problem of explanation for a markedly different kind of illness occurs in the relation of schizophrenia to social isolation: which is the cause, which the effect? The same problem occurs in the relation of schizophrenia to urban areas and social class. Schizophrenia is especially problematic because it belongs to that class of illness which is rather inadequately defined. Even though it is one of the better defined mental illnesses in comparison to the "psychoneuroses," its essential nature and cause and the most effective method for its treatment are all very poorly understood. And while a variety of studies all seem to agree that it is, compared to neurosis, comparatively common among the working classes and rare among the middle, the exact meaning of the finding remains obscure. The genuine contribution sociologists can make to the problem is likely to lie in demonstrating how deviants, some of whom may truly be psychotic, are nonetheless socially manageable and acceptable in some settings and not others. Eaton and Weil's study of the Hutterites[20] and Freeman and Simmons' studies of the relations of various family roles to the acceptability of deviance[21] are eminent cases in point. They do not attempt to diagnose or determine the etiology of illness so much as to study how and whether illness is recognized and how responses to it are organized.

Social Class Influences on the Responses to Illness

The most common approach to the problem of explaining the way people define illness and behave when sick has been predicated upon the reasonable assumption that what they believe, know, and value influences their behavior. A very large body of sociological and anthropological information has been collected about popular knowledge of and attitudes toward health and the institutions surrounding it, particularly in the United States. The greatest proportion of that literature is grossly descriptive, seeking to determine what people know and believe and how much of it accords with modern medical aims. The most exotic findings naturally come from studies of people who are submerged in an indigenous culture and have not been intensively educated in Western medical traditions. But by and large both anthropological studies using the idea of culture and sociological surveys of "popular knowledge" in industrial societies have been singularly vague. Aside from cultural designations like Mexican, Subanun, and Mashona, there is no method by which the material is ordered save for focusing on knowledge about *particular* illnesses. Such studies are essentially catalogues, often without a classified index.

In complex societies a very useful and popular mode of classifying behavior is offered by the idea of social class. However, it too requires more differentiation before its value can be fully exploited. Empirical studies have used as indices of social class, occupation, education, and income, individually or in combination. In addition to such elements there is also involved the element of class culture—the general style or pattern of thinking and behaving characteristic of some stratified segment of society, including patterns of distance and deference in relations between strata. Each element may have distinctly different bearing on responses to illness, but each tends to be confounded with the other under the term "social class." In the United States, class culture, level of education and information, and economic ability to pay for care are all prone to be confused; few studies have been able to distinguish clearly and instructively between economic opportunity and culturally and educationally motivated responses to illness. In countries where the class structure is relatively marked and traditional and its range wide, even with economic accessibility and level of information held constant, the mere pattern of deference holding between ranks and the position of the physician in the dominant classes may influence the inclination to seek care and the nature of the interaction between practitioner and patient.

The Organization of Responses to Illness

Careful sorting of the variables qualifying what people generally believe, know, and do about illness is necessary and useful as a way of understanding the social and cultural elements they bring to the process of being sick. But knowing the aggregation of elements brought to the process does not provide us with a way of organizing them. One way of organizing them is to recognize that the perception of and response to illness takes place over a course of time and that one can see it as a kind of career or cycle.[22] At the very least "illness behavior"[23] is problem solving in character, and we can speak of the various stages of perceiving a problem and the various attempts at solution. Recognition of this allows us to classify people's belief, knowledge, and custom by the priority of their introduction into the problem-solving process and by their bearing on estimating the period of time required for solution (or cure) and on the degree of recovery possible or expected. An additional source of organization lies in the fact that people who are ill are supposed to behave in ways appropriate to being ill. This is to say, being ill involves assuming a social role. Indeed, the concept of role seems to be the most important means by which we can develop a solid structure for our understanding of the behavior surrounding illness.

Talcott Parsons has given us a fairly refined delineation of the sick role.[24] He sees in the sick role one way by which deviant behavior and the response of others to that behavior can be organized. Biological disease may, of course, fall into the category of illness, as may forms of deviance with no apparent biological origin. The person defined as sick is relieved of everyday responsibilities, but he is also expected to take the proper steps in seeking competent help so as to be able to be cured and returned to normalcy. Defined as it is, the sick role is obviously a device for accommodating the behavior of others to the sick person and also for preventing the ill from withdrawing from society. Furthermore, it is a device for putting the ill in touch with therapeutic agents who can cure his deviance.

The nature of Parsons' contribution is of first importance, but the value of its substance is severely limited. The most casual observation indicates that what Parsons describes as the sick role has little relevance to much of the behavior surrounding illness. Some illness is not considered serious enough to warrant more than a slight reduction of everyday activity. Other illness is defined as incurable, to be adjusted to as such. Much illness never reaches the stage of formal consultation with a professional. Parsons' sick role obviously applies to only a small part of the process of seeking a cure for illness. Its limited reference to only some stages of the process of seeking help may be in part a necessary deficiency, however, for the earlier stages of illness, at which professional help is not yet prescribed and sought, are considerably less definite and thus more difficult to conceptualize with clarity.

A perhaps more serious deficiency in the idea of the sick role is its apparent inapplicability to populations other than those inclined to share professional values of universalism, achievement, and the like. From the approval with which it is used by both French and German writers, one might gather that Parsons' definition makes sense to middle-class Europeans as well as Americans. But working-class, peasant, and native populations, at least some of which are not inclined to use the professional consultant, are still left out. For them, being sick in a socially acceptable way does not hinge upon professional legitimation or even necessarily on special consultation with anyone.

What is needed is, in essence, specification of a set of roles corresponding to important and potentially final organized stages of the process of seeking help. This set of roles must include both permanent legitimate roles (like that of the "sickly" person, the handicapped, the mentally retarded),[25] temporary legitimate roles (such as "indispositions," female or otherwise); Parsons' sick role (which requires for its legitimation the pursuit of professional help), and both temporary and permanent roles to which moral stigma is attached even after the illness is to all intents and purposes "cured" (the mentally ill being the most outstanding case in point). Mental illness and drug addiction, as well as to a somewhat lesser degree mental deficiency, epilepsy, leprosy, tuberculosis, and venereal disease, are analytically interesting here precisely because many people cannot quite adopt a purely neutral "disease" orientation toward them; indeed, even when one is cured, the stigma remains in some sense to segregate the former patient from the normal and acceptable.[26]

I suggest, in brief, that it is necessary to construct a number of sick roles so as to be able to discriminate the characteristics of behavior expected from a person who is believed to have a minor, a major, or a fatal illness; a curable or an incurable illness; a short- or a long-term illness; and an ordinary or a stigmatized illness. With such a framework of possible roles we would have stable and significant points around which to order the particular and infinitely variable knowledge, belief, and customs to be found through time and across cultures. Furthermore, such roles focus attention not only on the sick person but also on those around him who urge him to behave in the properly sick way and on the consultant from whom he may be led to seek help. Of course, as soon as he is led to a consultant the sick person assumes the role of the client, or patient. An attempt at such sustained analysis now exists, though its empirical usefulness remains to be determined.[27]

The problem-solving activity of the sick person is composed in part of self-treatment, but often it is also composed of consulting others. Consonant with the rest of his analysis, Parsons' delineation of such consultation is restricted to formal consultation of a professional. The role of the patient is defined by reference to the behavior expected by the professional person. However, insofar as consultant roles need not be professional in character, the patient's role will vary correspondingly. The professional consultant's role is probably the most definite and stable of all to be found during the course of seeking cure, but there are other healer roles, all of which may be subsumed under the category "consultant." The career of seeking help may be seen to consist of initial self-treatment followed by the utilization of various lay and professional consultants. The variety of consultants has not yet been explored systematically, but it is certain that some are chosen precisely because they are *not* professional in character. The question some are asked is, "What would you yourself do, or what did you do, under these circumstances?" Thus, some are chosen as extensions of the patient's self, for their similarity and closeness to him, not their detachment. This consultant role, which involves little social distance from the patient and has its own distinct characteristics and functional limitations, can be contrasted to others that are characterized by increased social distance from the patient and require increasingly complex modes of organization in order to control the patient. The healer–client relationship may thus be seen as a function of the *particular* sick roles and healer roles that are in contact with each other. There is not *only* one relationship, and while it might be useful to consider the doctor–patient relationship prototypical as most writers do, Parsons prominent among them, that relationship itself varies far more than one might assume.

The Physician

From consideration of the sick role we are led directly to consideration of the consultant role and, through it, to the most definite consultant role of all, the professional in general and the physician in particular. The question for the sociology of medicine is how men are molded into physicians so as to be able to perform the healing role and what influences their performance once they play the role.

First, we may note that the prestige of physicians compared to other occupations is high in all industrial countries. Furthermore, the physician is the symbol of healing whose authority takes precedence over all others. In the United

States, the medical profession is the prototype of professionalism upon which all would-be healing professions model themselves. However, as has been pointed out rather trenchantly by Bucher and Strauss,[28] medicine is seen as a single profession at considerable expense of the facts. Within it are warring factions, each struggling for jurisdiction and control over various areas of work. The question is how, in spite of this variety of struggling "segments" within the ranks of those holding the M.D. degree and in the face of nonmedical occupations struggling for access to the task of healing, the profession still preserves a common identity and sustains a superordinate position.

Two sources of common identity are the greater visibility of the general medical degree over the special professional segments and the fact that the public's awareness is limited to the grosser, more symbolic aspects of the profession. Another source may lie in selective recruitment into the profession of people who are prone to share the same general outlook on work. Common social background may itself contribute to a certain homogeneity of outlook among doctors which significantly distinguishes them from people in such occupations as nursing and social work, who have typically more humble backgrounds.[29]

Significant as the background of physicians may be, however, it is likely to contribute only the bare bones of the professional medical outlook, for the would-be physician is a layman, lacking the knowledge to anticipate in detail the requirements for medical practice. The very fact that general practice, entrepreneurially organized, attracts many entering American medical students but progressively fewer as the years of training go on, indicates the erosion during training of a layman's idea of the proper type of practice. Medical school, like other professional schools, is supposed to have a profound socializing function. It is supposed to provide the student with the attitudes he needs to play the professional role properly and well. This socializing function of training has most preoccupied sociologists studying medical education.[30]

There is, however, a very real problem in assessing what medical school actually accomplishes and how many of its accomplishments are at once anticipated and approved by the faculty. There is no doubt that it imparts a great deal of technical knowledge and skill to its students, but there is ground for believing that the way doctors apply their skill not many years after graduation does not reflect the academic standards of their teachers.[31] Furthermore, one questionnaire study finds that, contrary to the faculty's intent, American students become "cynical," though other studies have qualified that finding.[32] An important participant–observation study indicated in some detail how students are led to restrict the level and direction of effort they make to learn what faculty members try to teach them.[33] And another study found that while the faculty seemed to have some influence on students' choices of medical speciality, it seemed to have virtually no influence at all on students' attitudes toward medicine as such.[34]

This evidence should not contradict the indubitable fact that doctors are not wholly born but are in some way made by medical school. The question is of detail and degree, and no very clear answer to it has as yet been offered. What does seem fairly certain, however, is that what the faculty believes to be true can be only partially so, and must be in part contradicted and counteracted by elements in the lay conceptions the student brings in with him and in the influence of his peers at school. Furthermore, members of the faculty must cancel out much of one another's influence, for like faculties everywhere, the medical school is broken up into departmental segments struggling for larger places on the curriculum and competing for the student's time, attention, and commitment. To be fully cognizant of such elements requires specific study of the medical faculty itself, a task that, aside from broad-scale treatments, has not yet been undertaken.

What evidence exists thus seems to indicate that fairly important elements in the training of members of the medical profession are not in fact consciously or rationally determined or controlled by the profession. The same may be said for an area that has received less attention than education—medical practice. If medical education molds the medical man, the exigencies of practice are likely to be the proof of the mold. It is for performing his role in the circumstances of practice that medical education prepares the physician. And it is in the realities of practice rather than in the classroom that we find the empirical materials for clarifying and articulating the actual rather than the imputed or hoped-for nature of the professional role. The question is, how stable and complete is the professional role in the face of the varied circumstances of practice, and if it is not entirely stable, which elements vary and which do not. Are doctors less "universalistic" in some forms of practice than others? Are they less functionally specific? In short, does their very professionalism waver in some settings?

Unfortunately, rather few systematic sociological studies of medical practice have been carried out, though much has been written on the topic. It would seem from historical materials that securing practice from extensive competition is one prerequisite for assuring stability. Furthermore, it seems plausible to think that the doctor's role will be closer to what is professionally desired when it is performed under the scrutiny of other doctors—in a hospital or a clinic for example—and when it may be carried out independently of lay influences. Hall's distinction between an "individualistic" and a "colleague" career[35] rests upon such criteria, as does Freidson's distinction between the client-dependent and the colleague-dependent practice.[36] These distinctions imply that the physician's behavior is at least in part contingent on the circumstances in which he practices. No study has as yet attempted to establish the degree of influence on professional behavior which may be exercised by lay clientele under certain conditions, but mere variation in prescribing habits is enough to suggest its strong likelihood, as is the adjustment of the professional's practice to patient preferences. Conversely, the influence of colleague groups on professional behavior is, under certain circumstances at least, patent. Coleman, Menzel, and Katz have indicated how integration into or isolation from a network of colleagues influences the speed of adoption of a new drug.[37] Seeman and Evans have indicated how medical care in one hospital varies with the qualities of the chief supervising physician.[38]

These findings suggest that perhaps a more realistic way to organize our knowledge about the behavior of the physician is to use the concept of professional role as a dependent variable. If the role is not completely stable and varies with the organized framework within which it must be exercised, the framework of practice itself might be the more appropriate unit to focus on. However, practice poses severe analytical problems. Unlike education and other mass services, medical care is difficult to organize into large, centralized social units. Social policy does indeed press for greater efficiency and lower cost, and physicians themselves are prone to desire convenient integration of services and facilities. But those centripetal forces are counteracted by the fact that medical care renders service to individuals who may require it quickly and at any hour, and so is stubbornly resistant to the centralization and integration into large-scale organizations common to most work today.

Medical practice is still characteristically and anachronistically practiced in a small, often one-man unit. Like its taxonomic cousin, the small, owner-operated shop, it poses the analytical paradox of being an organization without being a group, of being a unit distinct from its surrounding community, dependent upon being in some sense absorbed into the community. Difficult as it may be to conceptualize as an organization, however, the significance of the client and colleague group to the performance of the professional role requires attention to the practice in which they are encountered.

Other "Professionals" in Medicine

We have seen that the physician's behavior is not entirely accounted for adequately by the formal process of training supposed to mold him into a professional. Furthermore, we have seen that the milieu in which he practices plays some part in his performance. The milieu of practice, however, is not exhausted by reference to colleagues in medicine and patients. Increasingly prominent in the doctor's work are a variety of other occupations that come to form a complex division of labor in which medicine is dominant but nonetheless only a part. Those other occupations also have analytical interest for their bearing on the character of professionalism.

Of all such occupations, nursing has received the most sustained attention.[39] Thorner has analyzed the nurse's role in a way that implies it to be as fully professional as the physician's[40] even though there is great weakness in the position of the occupation. The nurse is typically subordinate both to the physician and to the hospital where she works. Furthermore, in spite of Nightingale's efforts in the nineteenth century, the nurse, because she is a female, has not been able to shake off the sexually rather than professionally determined mothering role. And the nurse's commitment to her occupation is not consistently and uniformly profound, for marriage is the aspiration of many and turnover is high. Indeed, like many others, the occupation is composed of a small proportion of policy makers, supervisers, and teaching nurses dedicated to professionalization, striving to mobilize a heterogeneous and shifting corps of often casual and transient skilled workers.

Pursuing the ever-present hope that schooling can in some sense influence the way the nurse sees herself and performs her role, studies that have been made of nursing students find that they do learn their lessons but that they also suffer from the incompatibility between their marriage and work aspirations.[41] Indeed, by pushing them toward a professional orientation, schools do not prepare them for subsequent subordination in the hospital, and so their lessons are understandably compromised in the face of reality. Perhaps the net effect of professionally oriented schools is to make the nurse more sensitive to her status, at once intensifying the normal inclination to pass on to lesser occupations one's "dirty work" and to require tactful treatment by superiors.

By and large, every analyst with the possible exception of those in nursing agrees that insofar as the concept of profession has any definiteness at all, the nurse is not fully professional. Like many other occupations in and around medicine in the United States, it is a would-be profession, and if only because of the strength of the medical profession is unlikely to attain full professional status. Its very struggle, however, and its claims, teach us something about the nature of professionalism and suggest that by attention to it and similar occupations we might be able to say much more about professionalism as an ideology and as a fairly recent social movement in modern society.

Most of these comments have relied on studies in the United States, which may not reflect very common issues elsewhere.[42] One issue certainly relevant elsewhere, however, is the relation of professionalism to the increasing necessity of technical training for work in industrial society. Such technical training could theoretically go on in unpretentious trade schools. The necessity to add the trappings of professionalism to what are essentially trade schools no doubt reflects in part both the necessity of attracting people with higher-than-artisan aspirations who have already had considerable general education and the complexity and responsibility of the tasks for which they are trained. Another important element, however, is the extent to which the trappings of professionalism can persuade the worker to become identified with his work in a way that mere technical training cannot. Identification with a job seems particularly important for those who, like some doctors and dentists, work isolated from colleague observation and supervision, but it is equally important as a device for motivating and controlling work in complex organizations, the most prominent of which is the hospital.

The Sociology of the Hospital

Several trends of analysis[43] may be perceived in the study of the hospital, some of which have direct bearing on professionalism. The relatively early studies of the hospital by sociologists were made with studies of the factory in mind, more particularly studies of the difficult position of the worker in that organization. In general, their view of the organization of hospital work could be summed up by the assumption—particularly characteristic of the "human relations approach"—that improving communication within and across the division of labor would settle difficulties of operation. The nurse being one of the earliest "workers" to be studied, the problem was to determine her needs, establish proper lines of communication, and sort out contradictory lines of authority.

A somewhat different point of view has been emerging more recently, emphasizing value conflicts, modes of discipline, and communication considerably less than the conflicting requirements inherent in the performance of varied tasks in the hospital, conflicts sufficiently objective that communication alone (rather than compromise, or the winning of a struggle) cannot solve them. There has been recent interest in approaching the organization by following out the implications of its frequently conflicting goals, the social requirements of the technical tasks being performed within it,[44] and the hospitals' sources of support. These studies have all contributed to the development of a considerably more sophisticated structural approach that, while perhaps less optimistic than the human relations approach, nonetheless seems to offer considerably more realistic promise in application. The hospital has also been used to test and refine more general hypotheses—such as that specifying direct relations between organizational size and administrative complexity. Perhaps more important, study has focused attention upon problems of analysis that have always been present in sociology but until now were rarely subjected to sustained examination.

The Professional in a Bureaucratic Setting

One such problem lies, on its simplest logical level, in Weber's analysis of rational–legal bureaucracy. As Parsons pointed out, Weber's analysis poses the problem of reconciling expert with hierarchical authority. Now, obviously, it is the *degree* of expertise that is at question, or else administration of any division of labor would be impossible. The expertise Parsons had in mind is the sort imputed to the professional: skill of such complexity and refinement that autonomy of judgment is necessary. Parsons suggested that Weber's monocratic model of rational–legal bureaucracy is an inappropriate work setting for the professional. An organization resembling a "company of equals" with only minimal hierarchical differentiation and supervision is instead the appropriate model. The university and hospital are cited as exemplary organizations, but no recognition is taken of the fact that, in the United States at least, both have well-developed bureaucratic administrations.

The early emphasis by Smith[45] on the "two lines of authority" in the hospital–administrative and medical–clearly implied the difficulty of operating such a system, while other writers more generally suggested that there were grave practical as well as analytical problems involved when professionals were to be found in bureaucratic organizations. Smith argues that those two lines of authority have unfortunate effects on the submedical staff because it is caught in the middle, but he does not indicate how both administrative and medical "authority" manage to coexist in the first place. However, Goss studied in some detail how autonomy of professional judgment could exist in a hospital setting that was patently hierarchical and supervisory. She observed that the two lines of authority are both established and maintained by the segregation of administrative decisions from areas where professional judgment was considered necessary, the former freely made and enforced by the authority of office, the latter left to the "authority" of the individual professional.[46] She further observed that hierarchical control in the professional sphere can be exercised by professionals of superior rank, but that it is done by means of giving advice rather than flat orders. On this foundation she constructed a model of organization variant from that defined by Weber, termed "advisory bureaucracy."

The value of Goss's distinction in other than logical ways remains to be seen. Is advice giving merely a form of etiquette in the United States, disguising an order that in other circumstances might be nakedly expressed? Is the pattern peculiar to the United States rather than characteristic of professional work groups everywhere? Similar observations must be made elsewhere before such questions can be answered, but what evidence exists implies that the pattern may be more American than general.[47] Nonetheless, in or out of the hospital, the analytical problem of the professional worker in formal organizations remains with us. And as a recent paper would have it, the use of the concept of bureaucracy may be entirely inappropriate for professional settings.[48]

The Motivation of the Nonprofessional Worker

Another organizational problem brought up by studies of the hospital is one of long standing. The alienation of the industrial worker from his work is a topic familiar to any reader of Karl Marx and sympathetic authors succeeding him. Industrial work is said to have become meaningless, dull, and dehumanizing. The worker tends to see his work as a source of income alone rather than of intrinsic gratification and important social identity. In spite of his alienation, however, mechanization, bureaucratic controls, and the incentive of wages in industry are more or less sufficient to control the quality of his work, if only because it requires so little commitment.

But the problem confronting the hospital is that much of the work it requires is not adequately performed when done mechanically and perfunctorily. This is particularly the case in the mental hospital, where the behavior of every worker in contact with the patient may influence his recovery. The problem becomes magnified further in the public mental hospital, where the patient is not a client but a ward, and so is more helpless, sociologically, than his illness alone implies.

Theoretically, the fully professional worker in the mental hospital poses no problem because he is committed to his work and finds both purpose and gratification in it; he may be trusted to behave therapeutically. Part of the problem with the nurse, of course, is that she is not fully professional; many methods have been developed to determine which nurses are the more professional and which the less. Professional or not, however, the nurse in American hospitals has delegated many of her tasks to even less professionalized workers so that, as in the prison, the personnel in continuous and intimate contact with patients are the least professional and of the lowest status. They are thus least likely to be committed to their work and may even be resentful of it. Furthermore, their characteristically lay perspectives are likely to contradict those approved by the hospital. And finally, their work is in part to hammer out a certain order and regularity on the wards. Consequently, they are prone to behave at best mechanically and unsympathetically and at worst punitively—in neither case therapeutically. They are said to behave in a custodial fashion.

A rather large literature has grown up around this topic, particularly in American state mental hospitals. The literature shows the characteristically American marks of a broad ideological emphasis on the intrinsic value of "democratic" rather than "authoritarian" relations. Attitude scales have been created purporting to measure "custodialism" and "humanism." Studies have been made of the influence on patient behavior of autocratic rather than permissive superordinates. Also relevant are studies of the worker's sense of status and opportunity for advancement, presumably factors giving dignity if not meaning to work.

By and large, the evidence supporting this approach is mixed and confusing. In some of the few precise studies of permissive leadership in medical settings, done under the direction or stimulus of Seeman, negative or ambivalent findings were characteristic.[49] Indeed, some of the evidence implied that the effects of permissiveness could be mischievous, increasing "communication" it is true, but also increasing mistakes. Furthermore, a study by Lefton and his associates implied that the new horizons opened to low-ranking hospital workers by a democratic ideology can make them less satisfied with their jobs than they were before.[50] And finally, with very few exceptions, these studies have taken place in the United States, where, culturally, there is strong pressure toward leveling the appearance if not the fact of difference in status and the exercise of hierarchical authority. Their findings may not apply to other settings where subordination is more traditional and acceptable.

The Organization as a Community

Coser's stimulating analysis of nurses deals with structural sources of the motivation to see oneself as an active, creative worker of some importance who can adopt a therapeutic rather than a custodial attitude toward the patient. This is the aim of all the studies just mentioned. However, few of them, including Coser's, have paid much attention to the fact that so long as it exists in its present residential form, the hospital will have inevitable custodial functions that someone must perform. The nature of such functions will vary from the hotel atmosphere of sanatoria like that described in *The Magic Mountain* to the prison-like atmosphere of the American state mental hospital, but they are both equally custodial. Indeed, the hospital, unlike the government bureau, the store, and the factory, is characteristically and taxonomically distinct as a residential, therefore custodial, institution. The question is, what are the consequences of being in custody?

A brilliant answer to that question has been suggested by Erving Goffman in his concept of "total institution," so named because it is in part a community and in part a formal organization. "A total institution may be defined as a place of residence and work where a large number of like-situated individuals, cut off from the wider society for an appreciable period of time, together lead an enclosed, formally administered round of life."[51] Mental hospitals, homes for the aged, concentration camps, boarding schools, and convents are all examples. Goffman notes that administration of the inhabitants of total institutions strains toward standardizing even the most intimate and personal activities by formally imposing on individuals grooming, dress, leisure, rest, and diet, uniform accouterments, and schedules. Standardization is not necessarily due to deliberate intent, but to very real needs for efficient utilization of administrative time, energy, and resources, and to the fact that by definition the organization is responsible for the well-being of the inmate and so cannot allow him to take responsibility for himself. The net outcome is the systematic destruction or at least repression of the former civil identity of the inmate. The inmate goes through a "series of abasements, degradations, humiliations and profanations of self." The process is intensified in the mental hospital by the rhetoric of imputing disease; whatever the patient may say or do can be described as a symptom and discounted as a responsible act deserving an answer on its own terms. In the face of this situation, one can understand the profound gap between those whose lives go on inside the organization and those who merely work there and live outside. Simply living inside encourages the development of an institutional culture, but in the face of the profound division between inmate and staff, it is a characteristically "inmate culture," oriented toward ways of evading and accommodating to the rules of the organization and the behavior of the staff.

The theoretical implication of Goffman's analysis is that a residential organization can under some circumstances come to be a community. Thus, it can influence the self even more profoundly than can other organizations. It is capable of stripping it of, even alienating it from, one identity and, as studies of small hospitals suggest, encouraging it to assume another. The implication of his analysis for psychiatry is that the best therapeutic intents cannot avoid custodial requirements that themselves damage the civilian identity of the patient and drive a wedge between him and those supposed to be helping him. Perhaps it was recognition of this fact that has led to experiments that eliminate custodial functions entirely by allowing the patient to reside outside hospital walls. Indeed, it is the community standing outside the hospital's walls that may be discussed now.

Health and the Community

There has been a fairly large amount of interest in ways of using the community itself as a therapeutic resource in the treatment and rehabilitation of the ill. Some indication of its effect on the course of illness and the fate of the sick person has been given by those who study how the mentally ill come to be hospitalized. The contrast between Eaton and Weil's study of a Hutterite community[52] and the Cummings' study of a Canadian community[53] indicates how variation in attitudes toward deviance can support the mentally ill and maintain them in the community or expel them from it. In a similar fashion, the predominant attitudes in a community can influence its acceptance and reintegration of the patient discharged from an institution.

But the community is not merely an aggregation of people or families which accepts or rejects certain illnesses. It is also composed of a network of organizations concerned with healing, only some of which are hospitals, clinics, or office practices. In the United States voluntary associations of patients or families joined together to help each other are especially interesting. In all industrial countries there are community agencies, whether of the state or of philanthropic societies, that provide services designed to help sick people. A few such agencies have received systematic study and Levine and White have suggested how their interrelationships might be conceptualized,[54] but the gaps in our knowledge about them are still profound.[55]

Finally, it may be noted that both the community and the agencies in it can be treated in a fashion that differs markedly from that used here. The analysis here has been of the behavior around disease and its management because it is believed that this represents what is distinctive about the sociology of medicine. Another orientation of great practical importance in medical affairs does not concern itself with disease so much as with the prevention of disease, particularly with changing the behavior and circumstances that are believed to cause disease.[56] In the form of "health education" this orientation seeks to persuade people to change their dietary, sanitary, child-rearing, and like habits, and adopt recommended practices. And in a form that has no definite label but that revolves around public health and social medicine, it is manifested in attempts to establish laws to enforce the maintenance of high health standards and to provide support to health services believed necessary for the population's well-being.

Medical Care—The Focus of the Field

In this short space I have covered a wide variety of topics connected with the field of medical sociology, some in a passing sentence, some in a paragraph, some in a page or two, but none in the detail each deserves. This is not the place for much detail. Here I have tried to sketch out the elements of the field only in order to provide a broad context for my focus in this book on medical care. That focus is, I believe, highly strategic, for it refers to the actual application of knowledge to human affairs, which is the pragmatic test of the meaning and consequences of everything else in the field. In the concrete settings of medical care—offices, clinics, and hospitals located in actual communities—we find coming together medical knowledge, the ideology of illness, the layman and his complaints, the physician and other workers. What goes on in those settings establishes the practical worth of the knowledge and research, the recruitment and training, and the status and rewards of the workers. The special position of the medical man is after all justified by his effective performance of practical ameliorative tasks, not by his contribution to abstract knowledge. It is in the character of its application to human needs that we find medicine's justification, and it is in medical care settings that application takes place. This is why I believe that it is more strategic to focus attention on the setting than on the other topics covered by the field of medical sociology.

Furthermore, I wish to argue that it is more useful to emphasize the organization of medical care settings than the attributes of their personnel—their training, devotion, and sensitivity. Indeed, in the next chapter I shall argue that medical sociology is badly in need of liberation from its reliance on the assumptions and concepts of the people it is concerned with, and in the chapter after that I shall try to indicate how the emphasis on organization—the "structural approach"—constitutes such a liberating force. It shall in fact be the approach of this book. Consonant with it, I shall not concern myself in any significant detail with the content of interaction between doctor and patient, or among doctors and other health workers. Instead, I shall focus on the significance of the way that interaction is organized by the formal, indeed often legal, relationships that establish the limits of legitimate behavior, and by the way in which the pattern of relationships exercises influence on the content of interaction independently of the individual characteristics of the participants. Such a focus requires that I emphasize the nature of medicine as an organized, dominant profession in an elaborate occupational and institutional division of labor, for at bottom it is that special position of the medical profession which seems to be at issue in the way medical settings operate. Only after fairly thorough exploration of such relatively abstract problems will it be possible for me to discuss the various settings in which medical care takes place and the prospects for improving their product in the future. That will end the book.

NOTES

1. Perhaps the only book that comes close to covering the whole array is constituted by a collection of papers written by a variety of authors—Howard E. Freeman et al., eds., *Handbook of Medical Sociology* (Englewood Cliffs, N. J.: Prentice-Hall, 1963). A revised edition is forthcoming.
2. David Mechanic, *Medical Sociology, A Selective View* (New York: The Free Press, 1968).
3. Eliot Freidson, *Profession of Medicine: A Study of the Sociology of Applied Knowledge* (New York: Dodd-Mead, 1970).
4. For bibliographies of anthropological studies see Steven Polgar, "Health and Human Behavior: Areas of Interest Common to the Social and Medical Sciences," *Current Anthropology*, 3 (1962), 159–205, and Marion Pearsall, *Medical Behavioral Science* (Lexington: University of Kentucky Press, 1963).
5. See, for example, Henry E. Sigerist, *On the Sociology of Medicine*, M. I. Roemer, ed. (New York: MD Publications, 1960); Richard H. Shryock, *Medicine and Society in America: 1660–1860* (New York: New York University Press, 1960); Vern L. Bullough, *The Development of Medicine as a Profession* (New York: Hafner, 1966); and George Rosen, *The Specialization of Medicine with Particular Reference to Ophthalmology* (New York: Froben, 1944).
6. *Current Work in the History of Medicine, An International Bibliography* (quarterly publication of the Wellcome Historical Medical Library).
7. See Freidson, *Profession of Medicine*, for a more extended discussion of illness as social deviance.
8. For example, William Rosengren, "Social Instability and Attitudes toward Pregnancy as a Social Role," *Social Problems*, 9 (1962), 371–378.
9. For example, Edwin Shur, *Crimes without Victims* (Englewood Cliffs, N. J.: Prentice-Hall, 1965).

10. Talcott Parsons, *The Social System* (New York: The Free Press, 1951), Chapter 10.

11. See, for example, Barbara Wootton, *Social Science and Social Pathology* (London: Allen and Unwin, 1959), and the discussion in Freidson, *Profession of Medicine*. See also Kingsley Davis, "Mental Hygiene and the Class Structure," *Psychiatry*, 1 (1938), 55–65.

12. J. L. Woodward, "Changing Ideas on Mental Illness and Its Treatment," *American Sociological Review*, 16 (1951), 443–454. See also Thomas S. Szasz, *Law, Liberty, and Psychiatry* (New York: Macmillan, 1963).

13. Kai T. Erikson, "Notes on the Sociology of Deviance," *Social Problems*, 9 (1962), 307–314.

14. D. C. Gilbert and Daniel J. Levinson, "'Custodialism' and 'Humanism' in Mental Hospital Structure and Staff Ideology," in M. Greenblatt et al., *The Patient and the Mental Hospital* (Glencoe, Ill.: The Free Press, 1957), pp. 20–35

15. B. Goldstein and Robert L. Eichhorn, "The Changing Protestant Ethic: Rural Patterns in Health, Work, and Leisure," *American Sociological Review*, 26 (1961), 557–565.

16. Arnold L. Green, "The Ideology of Antifluoridation Leaders," *Journal of Social Issues*, 17 (1961), 13–25. For a review of a large number of community decisions about fluoridation, see Robert L. Crain et al., *The Politics of Community Conflict: The Fluoridation Decision* (Indianapolis, Ind.: Bobbs-Merrill, 1968).

17. See the discussion in Freidson, *Profession of Medicine*, Chapter 13.

18. For a number of excellent discussions, see Duncan W. Clark and Brian MacMahon, eds., *Preventive Medicine* (Boston: Little, Brown, 1967).

19. See D. Hunter, *The Diseases of Occupations* (Boston: Little, Brown, 1957).

20. Joseph W. Eaton and R. J. Weil, *Culture and Mental Disorder* (Glencoe, Ill.: The Free Press, 1955).

21. Howard E. Freeman and Ozzie Simmons, *The Mental Patient Comes Home* (New York: Wiley, 1963).

22. For the idea of career, see Eliot Freidson, *Patients' Views of Medical Practice* (New York: Russell Sage Foundation, 1961). For the idea of a cycle, see B. Goldstein and P. Dommermuth, "The Sick Role Cycle: An Approach to Medical Sociology," *Sociology and Social Research*, 47 (1961), 1–12. For a more

elaborate treatment, see Charles Kadushin, *Why People Go to Psychiatrists* (New York: Atherton, 1969).

23. For an elaboration of the idea of illness behavior, see Mechanic, *Medical Sociology*.
24. Parsons, *Social System*.
25. For various "roles," see Thomas J. Scheff, *Being Mentally Ill* (Chicago: Aldine, 1966); Barney G. Glaser and Anselm L. Strauss, *Awareness of Dying* (Chicago: Aldine, 1965); Aaron Lipman and Richard S. Sterne, "Aging in the United States: Ascription of a Terminal Sick Role," *Sociology and Social Research*, 53 (1969), 194–203.
26. See Erving Goffman, *Stigma* (Englewood Cliffs, N. J.: Prentice-Hall, 1963).
27. Freidson, *Profession of Medicine*, Chapter 11.
28. Rue Bucher and Anselm Strauss, "Professions in Process," *American Journal of Sociology*, 66 (1961), 325–334.
29. See the discussion of medical values and the clinical mentality in Freidson, *Profession of Medicine*, Chapter 8.
30. See Robert K. Merton, "Some Preliminaries to a Sociology of Medical Education," in R. K. Merton et al., eds., *The Student Physician* (Cambridge, Mass.: Harvard University Press, 1957), pp. 3–79.
31. See the discussion of this and other matters in Samuel W. Bloom, "The Sociology of Medical Education," *Milbank Memorial Fund Quarterly*, 43 (1965), 143–184.
32. Howard S. Becker and Blanche Geer, "The Fate of Idealism in Medical School," *American Sociological Review*, 23 (1958), 50–56. See also the recent findings supporting the idea that "idealism" varies with the work setting: Robert M. Gray et al., "The Effect of Medical Specialization on Physicians' Attitudes," *Journal of Health and Human Behavior*, 7 (1966), 128–132.
33. Howard S. Becker et al., *Boys in White* (Chicago: University of Chicago Press, 1961).
34. R. E. Coker, Jr., et al., "Patterns of Influence: Medical School Faculty Members and the Values and Specialty Interests of Medical Students," *Journal of Medical Education*, 35 (1960), 518–527.
35. Oswald Hall, "Types of Medical Careers," *American Journal of Sociology*, 55 (1949), 243–253.
36. See Chapter 3 of this book.

37. See James Coleman et al., *Medical Innovation, A Diffusion Study* (Indianapolis, Ind.: Bobbs-Merrill, 1966).

38. M. Seeman and J. W. Evans, "Stratification and Hospital Care: I. The Performance of the Medical Interne," *American Sociological Review*, 26 (1961), 67–80, and M. Seeman and J. W. Evans, "Stratification and Hospital Care: II. The Objective Criteria of Performance," *American Sociological Review*, 26 (1961), 193–204.

39. For a recent selection of essays on nursing by sociologists, see Fred Davis, ed., *The Nursing Profession* (New York: Wiley, 1966).

40. I. Thorner, "Nursing: The Functional Significance of an Institutional Pattern," *American Sociological Review*, 20 (1955), 531–538.

41. For a recent study see George Psathas, *The Student Nurse and the Diploma School of Nursing* (New York: Springer, 1968).

42. A most essential work involving national comparisons is William A. Glaser's *Social Settings and Medical Organization: A Cross-National Study of the Hospital* (New York: Atherton Press, 1970).

43. The most comprehensive sociological treatise on the hospital is Johann Jürgen Rohde, *Soziologie des Krankenhauses* (Stuttgart: Ferdinand Enke Verlag, 1962).

44. For a review emphasizing technology and goals, see Charles Perrow, "Hospitals: Technology, Structure, and Goals," in James G. March, ed., *Handbook of Organization* (Chicago: Rand-McNally, 1965,) pp. 910–971. See also William R. Rosengren and Mark Lefton, *Hospitals and Patients* (New York: Atherton, 1969) and W. Richard Scott, "Some Implications of Organization Theory for Research on Health Services," *The Milbank Memorial Fund Quarterly*, 44 (October 1966), part 2, pp. 35–59.

45. Harvey L. Smith, "Two Lines of Authority: The Hospital's Dilemma," in E. G. Jaco, ed., *Patients, Physicians, and Illness* (New York: The Free Press, 1958), pp. 468–477.

46. Mary E. W. Goss, "Influence and Authority among Physicians in an Out-Patient Clinic," *American Sociological Review*, 26 (1961), 39–50.

47. Again, the work of Glaser is most relevant (see note 42).

48. Rue Bucher and Joan Stelling, "Characteristics of Professional Organizations," *Journal of Health and Social Behavior*, 10 (1969), 3–15.
49. Cf. Seeman and Evans, "Stratification and Hospital Care," I and II; John W. Evans, "Stratification, Alienation and the Hospital Setting," *Engineering Experiment Station Bulletin* No. 184, Ohio State University, 1960; and I. Oxaal, "Social Stratification and Personnel Turnover in the Hospital," *Engineering Experiment Station Monograph* No. 3, Ohio State University, 1960.
50. Mark Lefton et al., "Decision-Making in a Mental Hospital: Real, Perceived, and Ideal," *American Sociological Review*, 24 (1959), 822–829.
51. Erving Goffman, *Asylums* (Garden City, N.Y.: Anchor, 1961), p. xiii.
52. Eaton and Weil, *Culture and Mental Disorder.*
53. John and Elaine Cumming, *Closed Ranks* (Cambridge, Mass.: Harvard University Press, 1957).
54. Sol Levine and Paul E. White, "Exchange as a Conceptual Framework for the Study of Interorganizational Relationships," *Administrative Science Quarterly*, 5 (1961), 583–601.
55. For a recent attempt to sort out the relationships among the various agencies of the community, see Elaine Cumming, *Systems of Social Regulation* (New York: Atherton, 1968).
56. For a discussion of much material marked by this orientation see Edward Suchman, *Sociology and the Field of Public Health* (New York: Russell Sage Foundation, 1963).

Part 1

A SOCIOLOGICAL APPROACH TO MEDICAL CARE

1

The Present State of Medical Sociology

Some years ago Robert Straus made the useful distinction between an approach to the study of medicine which he called sociology in medicine and another which he called the sociology of medicine.[1] The distinction is important both conceptually and practically, for it includes within it the means of distinguishing what has been called social medicine in the past and what has grown to become over the past few decades a rather new approach to the area. The new approach is a potentially liberating one in that it can remove both medical knowledge and the practical arrangements for applying that knowledge to human affairs from the rather unhealthy intellectual and political isolation it has enjoyed over the past half-century, ever since medicine attained its present status as a dominant profession.

Essentially, Straus "suggested that the sociology of medicine is concerned with studying such factors as the organizational structure, role relationships, value systems, rituals, and functions of medicine as a system of behavior and that this type of [study] can best be carried out by persons operating from independent positions outside the formal medical setting. Sociology *in* medicine consists of collaborative research or teaching, often involving the integration of concepts, techniques, and personnel from many disciplines. . . . Research in which the sociologist is collaborating with the physician in studying a disease process or factors influencing the *patient's* response to illness are primarily sociology *in* medicine."[2]

In this book I shall examine medicine in general, but most particularly the medical profession and the institutions providing medical care from the point of view of the sociology *of* medicine. I shall attempt to show how, by adopting that point of view, one can better evaluate the nature of medical institutions in a way that is useful to the formulation of practical social policy. Indeed, I believe that only by adopting the perspective of a critical outside observer of medicine can one approach it in a way closely attuned to the public good, for while medicine has a foundation in scientific knowledge, its characteristics as a social institution lead it inevitably to have a distorted view of itself, its knowledge, and its mission. Collaborating with medicine in its institutionalized tasks requires adopting that distorted view with all its deficiencies. Studying it as an outsider allows one to see medicine as one of a number of human institutions, reflecting merely one of many intellectual points of view, one of many moral standpoints, and expressing the material interests and ideological commitments of only one of many organized groups in our society. Once one sees medicine that way, one is in a good position to evaluate how far social policy should allow the profession to determine for itself the terms of the medical care it provides the public, and how far not.

The Present Position of the Sociology of Medicine

The development of a sociology of medicine is a task that has barely been attempted in any serious and coherent fashion until recently.[3] The field itself is very new. It is true that the word "sociology" has been associated with medicine by one writer or another for many years. A book entitled *Medical Sociology* was published more than fifty years ago.[4] But the association was more one of good intent or rhetoric than of analytical significance. Until recently, the association of "medicine" with "sociology" meant merely that the writer believed that illness was not a purely biological phenomenon, that he recognized that social life formed the context for the practice of medicine, and that he was interested in the social and economic context of health and health institutions. But there were no distinctive concepts employed and usage was essentially unsystematic. For example, the stance of such a gifted scholar and admirable humanitarian as Henry Sigerist was essentially that of a humane physician with a keen eye for the social aspects of medicine. His marvelous analyses of tarantism and of homesickness[5] rested on his perceptive common sense, not on any special concept of illness, including that recognized by modern medicine, as a social construct.[6] And his trenchant and revealing commentary on the Hippocratic oath rested on his opposition to some of the conventional shibboleths of his guild, not on any special effort to arrive at some detached notion of the nature of medical practice.[7] This stance takes the essential premises of medicine for granted and seeks to reform medicine by showing that social factors play a part in it; the stance does not, however, seriously question or evaluate either the concepts of medicine or its conception of its place in human affairs. The approach is that of sociology *in* medicine.

Until recently, a sociology *of* medicine was not possible. Sociology had to become more a discipline than a brave program of positivist philosophers, and it had to develop tools of analysis as capable of dealing with the humble and concrete as with the grand. And the occupation of sociology had to grow to the point of producing trained practitioners rather than gifted amateurs. In fact sociology developed slowly over the nineteenth century, but its impetus gradually increased during the twentieth. The past several decades have seen marked developments in the discipline and the conditions of its exercise. Not many absolutely new concepts have been created, but many old ones have been refined and systematically elaborated. A tradition of empirical study developed and became routine. And the absolute number of trained sociologists has increased to the point where whole aggregates can focus on special areas of study and so begin the accumulation of information and awareness of problems which underlies a specialty. A reciprocal process has developed whereby general sociological concepts are applied to a special field and in the test of application are almost invariably found wanting. They are then reviewed, revised, and refined so as to be applicable to that special field and the revision is transmitted back to the mother discipline. On application to still other special fields, the concepts are revised more, in the hope of attaining at some time a dignified stability. However, while it has been prominent in many areas, this process has rather lagged in the area of medicine and health affairs.

The Underdevelopment of a Sociology of Medicine

Not until the 1950s were there enough sociologists interested in illness and medicine to reach the critical mass required for the development of a specialty. From then on, an increasing number of sociologists, including for a time some of the most prominent, began to think seriously about the character of illness, the doctor–patient relationship, medical education, hospitals, and other institutions of medicine. Indeed, aggregation of the interested proceeded at such a great rate that by the 1960s the newly formed Section on Medical Sociology of the American Sociological Association was about one-tenth the size of the entire association. It is in 1970 still one of the largest and most active sections. Number alone suggests that a full-fledged specialty had arisen in less than twenty years.[8]

However, the field has remained a specialty of number, a collectivity joined by vocational interest in the broad "medical" subject matter. Aside from somewhat greater experience in applying available methodological techniques to the collection of empirical data and a ritual use of jargon, sociological workers in the field have, with some exceptions, been largely indistinguishable from other workers. It is difficult to discern a distinctive approach to the area, a limited set of strategic concepts around which the entire range of phenomena may be ordered. The cause of this failure, I believe, lies first of all in the relatively weak state of sociology itself, which, even though strengthened markedly these past twenty-five years and encouraged by being fashionable in the popular press, has hardly arrived at the status of one of the physical sciences. But since all sociologists in every specialty share this burden, it does not help us to understand the special weakness of medical sociology. What seems to be peculiar to sociologists working in the field of medicine (including psychiatry) is an inordinate reliance upon the approach of the professional practitioners in the field and a distinct reluctance to use the approaches suggested by sociology itself. The emphasis is predominantly on sociology in medicine rather than on the sociology of medicine.

This medical rather than sociological orientation is demonstrated by the topics that have been studied intensively, by those that have been virtually ignored, and by the approach usually adopted toward the topics investigated. By far the most frequent topic studied is the health of given populations and its relationship to variables like age, sex, occupation, income, education, religion, and ethnic background. More sophisticated research in this area concerns itself with the concrete variables underlying or implied by those gross characteristics—dietary and other health-influencing customs, for example, or special types of environmental stress. By and large, both types might be called social epidemiology. From the point of view of the medically defined mission, they are very useful in measuring the extent of given health problems in the population, a task that is essential for determining what resources are needed by the health sector of the economy. Other studies focus on the utilization of health services, and to the extent that the administrative fact of utilization or nonutilization is the prime variable, to be associated with simple socioeconomic and demographic characteristics, these share the logic of epidemiological studies. In both cases the concern is with the distribution in a population of an attribute, trait, behavior, or experience that medical men believe to be important to the public good. Insofar as those attributes, traits, behaviors, or experiences are not themselves considered to constitute analytical problems to be studied critically, such studies do not provide concepts or information that allows the evaluation of what medical men believe or claim is important to the public good. Medicine may only be served, not evaluated.

Aside from studies of the correlates of illness and utilization, by far the bulk of remaining studies focus on various aspects of patient or prospective patient behavior. Here falls a rather large variety of analyses of the beliefs about and attitudes toward illness and the medical profession—studies of special ethnic groups in the United States, for example, or of relatively self-sufficient and exotic cultures in contact with Western medical institutions. Here also fall studies of the process by which people come to believe themselves sick and to seek some kind of care. The orientation of such studies varies a great deal, from those that consider the social behavior of the sick to be a unique area of study to those that regard it as at best a special instance of a more general class of human behavior, from common-sense correlation of social or administrative variables with simple attitudes to analyses employing systematic, sometimes specifically sociological, schemes.

The studies mentioned thus far are not only the most numerous in the field, but were also the first to be undertaken in any quantity as the field itself grew. What unifies them is their preoccupation with the layman as a social problem—whether or not he should be under medical treatment and, if he is not, why not. There is comparatively little concern with the extent to which it is not the layman but the physician, not lay but medical institutions, which are problems. There is typically what Roth calls "management bias."[9] And even when they are scrutinized, medical personnel and institutions tend to be evaluated from the point of view of medical norms.

It is of course easily understandable why most studies focus on the patient, for he is not only officially considered a social problem but also is more of a captive to the researchers than are other participants in the health care system. Similarly, it is no accident that in studies of health personnel, captives (which is to say students in nursing, dental, and medical schools, and post-graduate students in teaching hospitals) have been studied more often than full-fledged professional practitioners, and among practitioners the lower status aides and nurses have been studied more often than physicians.

By and large, I would argue, medical sociology has focused on the areas that the medical practitioner himself has considered problematic, adopting the conception of what is problematic from the profession itself without raising questions about the perspective from which the problem is defined. This is, of course, what one may expect from the point of view of sociology in medicine. In addition, I may say, even when sociological studies have turned their attention to the health worker himself, they have adopted the perspective of the worker in that they have emphasized the health worker's own conception of what is problematic about his own occupation and the other occupations with which he has worked. I refer here to a fairly exclusive focus on the attitudes of the worker—his personal commitment to his work and training, his professionalism, his conception of the patient—rather than on the way the worker's work is organized. This tendency is in part produced by relying on the survey questionnaire as the prime method of collecting data—an occupational disease of the sociologist that is present in all fields. But among sociologists of medicine, the tendency is accentuated by the primacy of a particular ideological emphasis in the field itself. The most prominent workers in the field of health are believed to be rather special kinds of people called professionals. By definition–and arbitrary definition–what is special about professionals is believed to be a stable set of ethical and other kinds of values which guide their behavior. The essential question asked is whether or not students have become professional by internalizing such values. Another question is whether or not attendants and nurses evidence such values and thus may be called professionals. In studies in this area, the tendency is not to question the value of the definition itself or to test its premise that professional behavior is contingent upon professional norms. Consequently, there has been little interest in studying the organized constraints upon individual behavior. Indeed, in the case of the physician we are extraordinarily ignorant of basic facts about the reality of medical practice–which is to say, the organization of medical care. Quite apart from the practical difficulty of study, part of that ignorance is a direct function of the assumption that attitudes and values –ethics and dedication–are more important than the circumstances in which they are tested. The assumption itself, while hardly illegitimate, is one espoused by the profession, which sees itself as a group with a special kind of knowledge and a special state of mind rather than as a group organized in a special way.[10]

In all, I would argue that while there are conspicuous and admirable exceptions, the bulk of the work of sociologists in the field of health has been medical and medical-professional rather than specifically sociological and independent in orientation. The premises underlying most work have been borrowed uncritically from the common sense of administrative policy, from the diagnostic categories of medicine, and from the ideology of the professional himself. The specialty of medical sociology has shown little of the ferment and independence now evident in the work of sociologists working in other areas, whether criminology, education, poverty, or other social problems. Why is this so?

Barriers to a Sociology of Medicine

Certainly one element explaining the sociologist's lack of detachment is his own humanity. He would be a poor human being indeed not to recognize the genuine suffering surrounding illness and the real value of much of modern medicine in ameliorating that suffering. In some instances the sociologist has deliberately assumed the role of a paramedical worker, cooperating in facilitating case finding and treatment as they are defined by current medical policy. The seductiveness of such ameliorative possibilities constitutes a distinct problem that sociologists in many other fields do not have to worry about, for in most other fields there are great differences of opinion about the proper way to manage a social problem and no one method of management seems clearly superior to any other. In medicine, on the other hand, a variety of resources is clearly related to the amelioration of suffering; there is simply not enough controversy about the central corpus of disease to lead to the questions that have arisen, for example, about the nature of crime. Furthermore, there is no room for doubt about the efficacy of medical techniques applied to that central corpus of diseases. No one can question the basic aim of health as one can question the aim of controlling crime by penal institutions. One might be for or against socialized medicine, but one cannot be for or against medicine itself; one might sympathize with the patient's unhappiness in medical institutions and explicate the attitudes, knowledge, and situations that contribute to his unhappiness, but one does not embrace folk medicine and reject modern medicine.

Clearly, medicine as well as the goal of health are relatively sacrosanct among present-day institutions. Sociologists studying factories, high schools, prisons, and other institutions are inclined to adopt an inquiring position when confronted with the lore of the people they are studying, seeking out the evidence, contradiction, and brute faith upon which the lore is based. But in medicine there has been less of such inquiry than there should be. There has been little critical inspection of the diagnostic and therapeutic customs that are brightened by the halo of "modern medical science" even though they have little connection with the basic knowledge of disease and the techniques by which it can be alleviated that is "modern medical science." Indeed, the halo effect of medical science itself extends not only to customs of management and practice but also to the way practice is organized. The sociologist, as an enlightened member of the professional classes, has faith in modern science and is led by the halo surrounding medical science to overlook the fact that generically the scientific knowledge of medicine has rather little relationship to the organization of medical care and that he is better equipped by his own knowledge than anyone else, particularly the physician, to analyze critically the organization of medical behavior and medical care institutions.

Furthermore, the sociologist himself tends to be apologetic and defensive about his own discipline. He aspires to have his discipline considered a science and to himself be considered a professional; to advance those aspirations he tends to take as his models the established sciences and the most secure professions. Since in the United States the physician is the professional par excellence, the sociologist may identify with him more than he is likely to identify with, for example, schoolteachers, nurses, factory workers, or other modest occupations. Indeed, he may identify with established professions more than is good for the practice of his own discipline.

Finally, most important, the field of medicine is so closely organized and the practice so autonomous that its study cannot be arranged easily. Permission to study medical settings and medical personnel may be granted by friendly administrators, but as all who have worked "in the field" know, administrative approval is but the first step of a successful study. To study patients one must obtain the permission of their physicians; to study physicians one must win their cooperation. Obviously, in both cases cooperation is likely to hinge upon the extent to which the proposed study conforms with the physician's notion of what "makes sense," what he himself is interested in and curious about, and what does not infringe upon his own prerogatives. Clearly, support and cooperation for a sociological study with other than a conventional medical view are not likely to be easy to obtain. In the United States physicians tend to control health and health-related institutions just as they tend to define the issues of public policy related to health (even though they do not control policy as such). The sociologist must enter the field by invitation, and even then only by the invitation of administrators and academics rather than practitioners. The invitation is framed by reference to problems that physicians themselves perceive. Without many sources of entrance independent of physicians, the sociologist's approach to the field will almost of necessity be influenced by his hosts and the topic of study limited to those settings to which access is gained.

These barriers to the development of a genuine sociology of medicine have been described rather starkly and over-simply in order to emphasize the degree to which the sociologist's work is dependent on and conditioned by the institutions he is supposed to be studying objectively. The situation existing for medicine differs only in degree from those prevalent in other fields. Whenever he ventures beyond arm-chair speculation and self-created research settings (as in his own classroom or in a laboratory) every sociologist is inextricably bound up in the institutions he studies. The sociologist working in the field of health is not uniquely but rather especially vulnerable to the danger of allowing the field he studies to define his problem for him.

Prime Tasks for a Sociology of Medicine

Taking into consideration the barriers to a genuine sociology of medicine and the limited development of the field thus far, what is to be done? There are many who are likely to feel that nothing need be done, if only because the lack of a special approach does not disturb them. Quite rightly, they emphasize the dignity and value of the approach of sociology in medicine, an approach directly related to assessing and formulating practical social policy in the contemporary field of health. But for those who are concerned with developing a disciplined understanding of human institutions independent of any single contemporaneity, any ephemeral Establishment, the approach of sociology in medicine is not enough. What must be done is to formulate a consistent way of thinking and ordering data that is independent of the institution studied and therefore applicable to many institutions in many times and places. I would argue, however, that such an approach is not "merely" theoretical. If it is successful, it becomes a far more useful instrument for formulating social policy than an approach rooted in medicine itself. By the very fact of being detached from medicine the approach allows social policy to examine medicine and medicine's claims as one of a more general species, and thus to evaluate better the relation of its needs and claims to those of other professions. Furthermore, insofar as it attempts to develop precise concepts general enough to apply to more than the present-day profession in the United States, the sociology of medicine can provide a much more sophisticated and useful guide to long-term planning of social policy than the approach that is limited to the point of view of the present-day institution of medicine.

What are the tasks of such a sociology of medicine? A number may be mentioned here, but in performing all of them one quality should prevail: the sociology of modern medicine should adopt the same detachment and suspension of commitment that it is inclined to adopt in the study of folk or primitive medicine. Taking as little as possible to be self-evidently true in what the profession claims for itself and its institutions, it should be obliged to develop an approach relying on data that are relatively independent of those claims. Such data lie not in expressed attitudes and opinions but in behavior, and—most especially for sociology as a discipline distinct from psychology—in the organized patterns of behavior called institutions or organizations. Such organized patterns of behavior may be treated as something separate from any individual participating in them and may be seen to influence the behavior of the participating individuals. As I shall note in the more extensive discussion of the next chapter, it parallels the approach of ecology by emphasizing the influence of environment in limiting the possibilities of individual behavior. In the context of the sociology of medicine the approach is, I believe, one that virtually assures an analytic stance distinct from that of medicine: it eschews the characteristic emphasis of medical science on the biological processes taking place within the individual organism and the characteristic common-sense individualism that lies at the heart of the approach of the medical profession to itself, its practices, and its relation to patients. While I do not believe that this structural or environmental approach is the only legitimate one or that it is useful for all purposes of analysis, I do believe that it is especially useful for adopting a stance independent of the profession under study.

Another essential task required of a sociology of medicine is performed by using that structural approach to formulate concepts that can delineate both the profession and its institutions in terms independent of the profession's own ideology. The profession must be seen not merely as a collection of individuals trained in a particular way and possessing certain ethical standards, but as an occupation organized in a particular way, with stable relations to other occupations and standing in a particular relationship to its clientele. In essence, it must be seen as a status in society, participating in a division of labor and in given organizations. And the behavior of its members can be seen as a product of those structural relations. Given this orientation toward the profession, the formulation of social policy certainly requires preoccupation with recruiting and training practitioners and with the modes by which they will be compensated for their services. But it also requires concern with the organization of a larger division of labor in which the profession is but one member, the jurisdictional and other relations of many occupations each to the other, the place of the various occupations in the institutions of practice, the support of occupational prerogatives, and the legal reinforcement of the authority of the practitioner over his clients. These structural characteristics can be understood independently of recruitment and training, and once we understand them, many practical policy issues can be managed largely by changing the legal and administrative framework without the necessity of undertaking the difficult task of attempting to change individuals' values and attitudes directly.

A sociology of medicine must also develop orderly ways of analyzing and evaluating the way the profession's work is organized and performed. Given the framework provided by delineating the nature of the profession, the task is to develop a method of analyzing the organization of its work with concepts analogous to those used in industrial sociology to delineate the factory, plant, or industrial enterprise. Here again, the issue is not the attributes of the individuals involved so much as the way in which all individuals' relations each to the other are ordered by the organized set of positions in the enterprise.

Finally, it seems necessary to develop a method of dealing with the knowledge and practice of the profession in such a way as to be able to examine it as but a member of a more general social class of knowledge and practice, independent of the point of view and persuasion of the profession and its clientele, and without commitment to the time and place in which the profession is being studied. In the case of medicine, this task revolves around the analysis of the nature of disease and of the medical science and practice addressed to it. Of necessity, solution is not gained by adopting the particular point of view of the profession itself, but rather must be gained by adopting an independent stance that rests upon the point of view generic to sociology, that sees all knowledge and practice as being essentially social creations rather than physical facts. With such a solution, the analytical tradition of the sociology of knowledge seems the most appropriate tool.

Toward a Sociology of Medical Care

In this book I wish to suggest in some detail how some of the tasks prerequisite to the development of an adequate sociology of medicine might be performed. I do not plan to attempt all the tasks, but rather, after some general review of the field, to attempt only those related to the study of the way medical care is organized. The organization of medical care is considered to be the central issue for a sociological analysis of medicine. It is central because, I argue, the organization of the activity places limits on what can go on in social life. It is the organization of health services that determines how those services are presented and carried out by physicians and other workers. And it is the organization of health services that gives shape, substance, and meaning to the experience of the patient seeking and receiving those services.

I shall try to create a framework within which the organization of medical care can be seen more clearly. I shall first attempt to specify the nature of the structural approach I adopt, partially anticipating in my discussion some of the ways I shall examine health services. Given a specification of the approach, I shall undertake a series of discussions to suggest some of those critical features of the profession which dominate the provision of health services. After a general overview of the characteristics of the profession, I shall concern myself with those structural features of the profession that seem to determine the distinctive character of health services, and the quality of experience that laymen obtain in the course of receiving health services. Finally, I shall attempt to indicate the relevance of the concepts created by my approach by discussing some concrete programs designed to explore new ways of providing health services, and I shall evaluate them from the point of view of the concepts of the sociology of medical care.

NOTES

1. Robert Straus, "The Nature and Status of Medical Sociology," *American Sociological Review*, 22 (April 1957), 203.
2. *Ibid.*, p. 203.
3. For reviews of the content of the entire field, see H. E. Freeman, S. Levine, and L. J. Reeder, eds., *Handbook of Medical Sociology* (Englewood Cliffs, N. J.: Prentice-Hall, 1963); Steven Polgar, "Health and Human Behavior: Areas of Interest Common to the Social and Medical Sciences," *Current Anthropology*, 3 (April 1962), 159–205; and the Introduction of this book.
4. James P. Warbasse, *Medical Sociology: A Series of Observations Touching upon the Sociology of Health and the Relation of Medicine to Sociology* (New York: Appleton, 1910).
5. Henry E. Sigerist, "Science and History," in *Lectures on the Scientific Basis of Medicine*, Vol. 3 (London: University of London Press, 1955), pp. 1–16.
6. An attempt to create such a concept is found in Eliot Freidson, *Profession of Medicine* (New York: Dodd-Mead, 1970), Part 3.
7. Henry E. Sigerist, *Medicine and Human Welfare* (New Haven, Conn.: Yale University Press, 1941), pp. 105–145.
8. For a brief history of medical sociology and its growth, see Howard G. Freeman, Sol Levine, and Leo G. Reeder, "Present Status of Medical Sociology," in Freeman et al., *Handbook of Medical Sociology*, pp. 473–491.
9. Julius A. Roth, " 'Management Bias' in Social Science Study of Medical Treatment," *Human Organization*, 21 (Spring 1962), 47–50.
10. For a sustained critique of this concept of profession, see Freidson, *Profession of Medicine*.

2

A Structural Approach to Medical Care

As I pointed out in the last chapter, the approach of the sociologist *in* medicine is quite properly the approach of medicine itself. This approach, like that characteristic of our times in general, is individualistic in character, for we have been in the age of the psychological man.[1] The tendency of everyday thought is toward what might be called "common-sense individualism." In the case of medicine, the orientation of common-sense individualism carried over from lay habits of thought is intensified even further by medicine's characteristic preoccupation with the human being as a discrete, individual organism. The organism can be seen as an environment for microorganisms, perhaps, and as influenced by the traumatic or infectious charac-

This chapter is a revision of an address given at the Symposium on the Cultural and Social Environment of Man and Its Significance for His Biological Performance, School for Advanced Studies, Downstate Medical Center, State University of New York, April 27, 1967.

teristics of the environments in which they are to be found, perhaps, but always with a certain self-sufficient integrity of its own. Bodies are not seen as functions of the environment but rather as influenced by the environment. The individual body is the prime unit of analysis. Furthermore, the individual is the prime unit of explanation in that his performance is explained by the way in which his body and "mind" function, for example, by his physical impairments and his intelligence or motivation. Thus, the "illness" of the patient is explained by the characteristics of the disease entity found in him, and the disease is treated to remedy the difficulty.

The approach of many sociologists *in* medicine to the problem of providing medical care to the sick offers the same common-sense individualism. In that area, the approach is reinforced by the characteristic individualism of the medical view of disease, and more particularly by the ideological individualism of the profession's view of itself and its work. The professions in general and the medical profession in particular tend to see themselves as creative self-regulating individuals more than a few cuts above ordinary humanity. In considering how the members of the profession work, its leaders typically see solutions to the problem of poor or unethical work in recruiting better-motivated and more capable entrants to school, in improving their professional education, and in generally "raising standards." All these devices are predicated on the aim of changing the quality of *individuals*, the assumption being first that social pathologies connected with medical care, like illnesses connected with mankind, are "caused" by the characteristics of the individuals providing the care rather than by the environment in which those individuals provide care, and second that they are best treated by treating the individuals rather than the environment.

In this chapter I suggest that by adopting the view of common-sense individualism we severely handicap the possibility of attaining both our moral and practical ends. I want to outline another approach to analysis and practice, one that does not have to make the assumption that there is such a thing as individuality but that, paradoxically, creates the conditions for a richer individuality than pursuit of the individualistic approach allows. If we must assign a label to this alternative mode of thinking about medical care, the sociological term "social structure" is useful. The term implies a perspective that is by no means foreign to anyone familiar with the theory of evolution and the principles of ecology. Indeed, the mode of reasoning contained in the idea of social structure is quite similar to that in the theory of evolution.

Environment and Survival

The key variables specified by the theory of evolution are (1) the finite quantity and forms of energy or resources available in a given environment, (2) the capacity of a species to use available resources, and (3) the fate (i.e., expansion, maintenance, reduction, or disappearance) of the species. A species will survive insofar as it is well adapted to utilizing the resources of a given environment. Insofar as some individuals in a species are better adapted than others to utilize the resources of a given environment, they are more likely to survive than others, and, assuming their adaptation can be transmitted genetically, they will shape the species of the future.

By reference to the limits of the environment and the characteristics of species, the theory of evolution attempts to explain how species come to develop and subsequently thrive or die out. The critical analytical element is the environment, which sets limits on the number and types of organisms that can survive. Given random variation among individuals, it is the environment and the niches it offers that determine which individual will thrive. By the same token, the energy available to a given niche determines how many individuals can survive in that niche, and how comfortably. The environment for any individual, of course, is not only energy in one form or another but also other individuals competing for the usable energy available. Thus, *the environment may be seen to shape the species*, the behavior of the species that survives being a function of the environment. One need not assume any motive or aim or impulse on the part of the species save that of survival. What survives and thrives is that which happens to be adapted to the environment. One can predict what will happen to a species from the environment.

I hope it is clear from this description how unimportant are the ideas of individuality and individualism. One can use the characteristics of the environment to predict the nature of the species that will survive or the changes that must occur either in environment or in life in order for life to survive. Neither individualism nor individuality is denied —they are simply tangential to the central idea of the constraining environment and the necessity for adaptation by the species.

This admittedly oversimple sketch of the mode of thinking characteristic of the theory of evolution is presented as a kind of foil for contrasting the common-sense view of contemporary social life that underlies much writing about medical care. Instead of seeing it as an environment within which individuality occurs, social life is seen as a product or consequence of individual characteristics. Instead of concern with creating environments that encourage one kind of adaptation rather than another, there is concern with creating adaptations out of whole cloth, independently of the environment. These emphases are as characteristic of medical as of other social policy and, I would argue, are not theoretically sound, practically useful, or morally good.

Individual and Structural Explanations

Our civilization emphasizes choice over constraint, the individual over the group, and the actor over the environment. In reflecting that emphasis, our legal, religious, and educational institutions, even our scientific institutions, reflect a moral value which is, I believe, worth honoring. However, to assign moral value to the individual over the environment is not the same thing as to explain how individuals become what they are or to undertake a realistic program of changing individuals. It is one thing to hold a value and quite another thing to decide how to act so as to attain that value. I believe our moral preferences have so conditioned our way of looking at the world that we have come to confuse them with the way the world works. We have been led to see the world intellectually in a fashion that is neither elegant nor economical nor useful. Indeed, our moral preferences have led us to overemphasize ways of changing the world that are actually highly destructive of what we value.

Essentially, our instinct is to analyze the human world by reference to individual motives, values, and knowledge rather than by reference to the organization of the human world itself. Thus, in attacking what is wrong in the world our inclination is to emphasize what is wrong in the individual and pour our efforts into ways of changing the individual rather than his environment. And so it is that we emphasize clinical medical treatment, psychotherapy, and education in our ameliorative programs, all in the hope of improving individual lives and performances. Like most Western religions, we are prone to try to change the world by changing men's souls. We tend to see the world as composed of a multitude of individuals whose actions are a function of the free choices they make, choices limited by the individual's faulty education, poor health, personal maladjustment, or inadequate religious commitment. Individual behavior is a function of individual imperfection. It follows that if we can change the individuals of our world by improving their education, their health, their emotional balance and personal insight, and their religious or moral commitment, we can bring the millennium.

Such common-sense individualism characteristically makes two flawed assumptions. The first is that since the human world is made up of individuals there is no such thing as a relatively stable, structured, social environment that constrains, limits, and channels an individual's behavior regardless of his personal qualities. That assumption, however, is simply empirically untrue. Granted that in the last analysis groups are indeed composed of individuals and therefore exist only through individuals, to any concrete *given* individual, the aggregate of other individuals with whom he is in interaction constitutes an organized social environment independent of him. Both the social and the physical environments limit the resources and opportunities for choice available to him quite independently of his own individual desires and capacities.

As in ecology, the organization of all species in a given environment limits what is available to any single species. Within any single species the absolute number of individuals in relation to the quantity of resources limits what is available to any single individual. Due to its individual qualities one organism may be able to get more of the available resources than another, and therefore thrive *compared* to another, but the outcome is still absolutely limited by the resources available. Taking all the individuals together, we find that the *average* outcome possible for the individual is a function of the environment, while variation about the mean or average may be a function of individual difference. The mistake our common-sense individualism makes is to confound individual performance with the *average* of performance. It ignores the role of the environment in creating the average, which is to say limiting the absolute magnitude of high and low performance by individuals. Individuals do vary, but taking an aggregate of individuals, they vary around a mean or average. The environment can be seen to limit the mathematical value of the mean and the absolute limits of variation around it. Individual differences may be seen to underly variation above and below the mean.

The second flawed assumption of common-sense individualism is that the individual's characteristics are definitely formed at some point of time into a stable and fixed bundle of knowledge, motives, and values, and that therefore he will act, from that time of formation and subsequently, more or less the same way no matter what the environment he acts in may be. That is, we are prone to assume that socialization during childhood, religious conversion, professional education, and intensive psychotherapy—all distinct and segregated events, limited in time—have such permanent and significant influence on the individual that they will determine how the individual will behave in any subsequent environment. This assumption justifies the effort involved in changing individuals—after all, if cure lasts but a day, why bother?

Nonetheless we fly in the face of available evidence in believing that a critical and discrete event or process can so firmly mold the individual as to mark him for life as well as to determine the kind of choices he will make subsequently, no matter what his environment. We "test" this flawed assumption not by examining the behavior of the majority or the average, but rather by citing the inspirational exception. In our *Readers' Digest* minds, we attend to the extraordinary persons in whom a religious conversion, experience with a great teacher, or a profoundly moving psychoanalysis produced a new man indelibly, for all subsequent life. Honest testing of the validity of the assumption is simply ignored; it is conveniently forgotten that the *average* person is at best only mildly influenced, independently of his social environment, by his education, his religion, or his psychotherapy.

The structural approach of sociology makes none of these dubious and obscurantist assumptions. Its assumptions are rather simple. First, it assumes that whatever motives, values, or knowledge people have come into contact with and have "internalized," they do not guide the behavior of *most* individuals unless they are continually reinforced by their social environment. Second, the approach assumes that the environment can, by reinforcement, lead people to forsake one set of motives, values, or knowledge in favor of another. And third, given the first two, the average behavior of an aggregate of individuals can be predicted more successfully by reference to the pressures of the environment than by reference to the motives, values, and knowledge they had before entering the social environment. The basis of prediction is from the requirements for social "survival" posed by the social environment and refers to the functional adaptations of the aggregate of individuals who survive. Prediction is, of course, statistical, inapplicable to any individual except as a probability value.

Social Structure and Medical Policy

I hope that by now I have succeeded in making clear the distinction between analysis of human behavior by reference to the qualities and capacities of individuals and analysis based on the influence of the social environment in limiting what an aggregate of individuals can do and still survive. And I hope that in the latter case the parallel with the thinking characteristic of the biological theory of evolution is clear. Certainly I have had to be rather vague and general, but since I now want to use these distinctions to discuss medical policy, perhaps they will become somewhat more definite.

In brief, I wish to suggest that in our approach to problems of *individual health* our thinking has been dominated by the common-sense individualism I have described. Consonant with the bias of medical thinking, medical policy has emphasized the clinical treatment of individuals well past the boundaries of prudence and good sense. Furthermore, in our approach to problems of the provision of clinical health services, uncritical common-sense individualism has been prone to emphasize almost wholly the importance of the formal selection and education of individual practitioners rather than the social environment of practice.

I do not wish to dwell on the first problem very much, but it is worth mentioning. In our war on illness we have typically adopted common-sense individualism and emphasized "educating" the layman to avoid illness-producing situations. When he becomes ill and approved first aid has failed, we have tried to lead him to seek out a licensed practitioner and cooperate with his regimen. The burden of responsibility is on the individual to avoid illness or, if he does become ill, to behave properly in seeking help. Rather little concern is devoted to the illness-producing situation itself save by those lonely minorities in public health and preventive medicine to whom academic medicine gives virtually no respect or prestige.

Think for a moment of analogies to this emphasis. Imagine building housing without fire escapes, fire retardant materials, or sprinkler systems. Instead, reliance is put on educating the public to be careful with matches and small boys and on teaching them where plastic surgeons can be found when small boys succeed and first aid fails. Public figures deplore the shortage of plastic surgeons and the Burn Foundation has a March of Dollars so as to be able to pour resources into improving clinical knowledge about burns and into caring for the indigent burned. Social policy focuses on "educating" prospective patients and grinding out enough physicians or physician-substitutes in order to serve the large number of patients who were not successfully educated.

Take another example. Imagine building roads so as to virtually encourage collisions by all but the unusually alert, rational, self-controlled, and lucky, and building automobiles that contribute to rather than protect from the trauma of collision. This individualistic policy focuses solely on "safe driver" education programs, on increasing the supply of well-trained orthopedic surgeons to handle the failures of education who suffer a collision, and on improving the clinical treatment of the consequences of accidents.

These examples do not illustrate merely the strength of organized economic interests, the weakness or indifference of political authority, and the self-destructive selfishness of the taxpayer. They also illustrate a perspective on the world that sees the solution of human problems in educating individuals and, where necessary, treating individuals, but rarely in changing the individual's environment to prevent the likelihood of the problem arising in the first place. It is each individual who must watch out for matches, overloaded wires, overheated stoves, flammable materials; who must stop, enter with caution, watch the other, keep distance, stay sober and awake.

Medicine's emphasis on clinical practice represents the same perspective, an outpouring of great energy and creativity into the very real problem of individual therapy and patient education but virtually no energy or ingenuity devoted to attacking the considerably more direct problem of the environment. Given the serious and complex issue of the degree to which preventive and therapeutic use of the environment may interfere with individual freedom, surely much more can be done, surely the burden of the environment could be lightened so as to avoid the necessity of clinical treatment.

But as I said, therapy for specific disorders is not my prime concern. My concern is the social environment represented by the social structure and I wish to focus on human behavior unconnected with biological illness. The social structure is less salient to biological illness than to the response of patients and physicians to illness and the effectiveness with which that illness can be identified (or diagnosed) and treated. Critical to the treatment of illness, of course, is the performance of the physician. In considering the problem, conventional solutions have emphasized medical education. I want to discuss the problem from the point of view of social structure. I want to suggest how the environment created by the organization of medical practice encourages the doctor to behave one way rather than another.

Social Structure and Medical Care

Traditional management of the problem of assuring an adequate standard of medical care consists of recruiting intellectually capable medical students, training them properly before licensing them, and then turning them loose to practice. Such management rests on untenable assumptions about the stability and strength of motives, values, and knowledge absorbed within the course of a limited period of formal education. Furthermore, I suggest, the present organization of medical practice systematically encourages the *average* physician to give indifferent medical care. (I am not talking about the extraordinarily successful physician, academic or otherwise, but about the *average* physician who is, like most men, neither devil nor saint.)

Consider the way medical practice is organized among such primary care medical workers as general practitioners, pediatricians, and internists.[2] They generally work in their own offices, rented and furnished by their own capital, usually alone but sometimes with a compatible colleague or two. And they must pay the rent and support their families like anyone else. They obtain the money they need from individual patients who have submitted to their care, and their economic support increases directly with the number of patients who seek help from them and the number and type of services they give to patients.

Now how is such a practice "built"—that is to say, how does a physician establish himself in his niche, survive, and even thrive? He builds his practice by pleasing one patient, who tells his friends, pleasing the friends who tell *their* friends, and so on. Here is both the blessing and the curse of solo fee-for-service practice—that when the supply of practitioners is ample enough to force competition for patients, the practice thrives by pleasing the patient. The blessing lies in the sense of security and the catharsis the patient obtains. The curse lies in the technical quality of the care that will in fact please patients. Surely much of the excessive prescribing of antibiotics, barbiturates, tranquilizers, and other drugs must be ascribed to pleasing the patient or to giving in to him out of sheer weariness. And these prescribing practices, drawn into public view by the fact that a manufactured article is involved, must represent merely a fraction of the dubious but less visible ways the primary-care physician is led to please his patients.

In addition to providing an environment in which the average primary-care physician is encouraged to give patients what they want whether or not it is clearly indicated medically, the organization of solo fee-for-service private practice insulates him from colleagues who might otherwise stiffen his resistance to "giving in" to the patient. Furthermore, colleagues are not there to question his self-deceptions. It is doubtful that the average physician knowingly employs questionable practices. Isolated from others, he simply comes to believe that his poor records, shortcuts, and readiness to prescribe are all harmless and insignificant practices. Insulated from day-to-day face-to-face interaction with colleagues, he meets no important pressure of opinion opposed to that of his patients, and none to warn of danger or impropriety. In a situation like this, how sensible it is to believe that he will practice the way he was taught in medical school, let alone learn and use the new knowledge and techniques discovered subsequently? What evidence is available from the United States and Canada suggests that in this situation the quality of performance declines over the years.[3]

The primary-care practitioner—the general practitioner, the pediatrician, and internist to whom patients come on their own initiative and on the referrals of friends rather than of other physicians—is the traditional prototype, the ideal image of medical practice. But there are other kinds of practitioners often called specialists who are more closely linked to colleagues than patients by virtue of depending on colleague referrals rather than patient choice. In the solo fee-for-service system, however, their major link is with the primary-care practitioner.

Here the significant pressure on practice is clearly that of the referring physician, for as the "feeder," the referring physician's satisfaction with the way his patient is treated is crucial to his decision to refer subsequent patients. The feeder, who is himself under pressure from his patients to conform to their conceptions of therapy, exerts pressure on the man he refers to. If the specialist works alone, his work is visible only to his feeders and contingent on their approval. He is thus in much the same position as his feeders, though, since his feeders know more medicine than do patients, pressure may not be of the same quality. But his feeders do not know as much about his specialty as he and may exert ignorant but nonetheless powerful pressures. The strength of this pressure on his performance is particularly great when there is no need to hospitalize the patient or when, if hospitalization is needed, the hospital privileges of the attending physician are well-nigh absolute. In both cases, pressure to deviate from academic standards of practice is unopposed by countervailing pressures from colleagues. Quality is unlikely to be academic. Here again the *situation*, not the *individual*, is critical.

In this sketch of the conventional structure of medical practice in the United States I have had to oversimplify by ignoring variations in organization as well as in the supply of physicians and the structure of supervision in hospitals. Details must wait for later chapters. Here I have merely seized on some of the common elements of the system and tried to show how they operate to systematically influence medical care regardless of the qualities of the individual physicians involved. What evidence there is indicates that the immediate organizational environment of practice influences performance more than such things as the personality or education of individuals. By and large, I would argue, it is difficult to think of a worse way of organizing the practice of medicine than the traditional method I have described. The major pressures of the system are directed toward increasing the number of services and decreasing the professional quality of those services. Such a system of organization is predicated on the assumption that a properly equipped man will perform at his best regardless of his environment and that our prime job is to equip him properly. This is, I insist, an untenable assumption.

The Average and the Exception

It is very important to keep in mind the fact that there are two ways of measuring the consequences of a social system. I have devoted myself to the consequences for the *average*—the majority of the profession that is so inconspicuous to medical policy makers, those without teaching hospital affiliations or even any hospital affiliations at all, most if not all of whose time is spent seeing patients in private offices. These are the people who give most of the care to most of the patients most of the time, and these are the people who become what the structure of practice urges them to become. These are the ones for whom the social structure is too great a burden.

However, defenders of solo fee-for-service private practice argue to the average man as little as do the defenders of a free market system. In the latter case, after all, the average entrepreneur is the near-bankrupt desperate small-business proprietor who must work himself and members of his family harder and longer than he could work employees, and at less pay, to gain mere survival. Nor do the defenders of either system argue to the failures—the businessmen who go bankrupt and the physicians drawn into shady or shabby practices. Both argue to only one tail of the normal distribution—the extraordinary success, the great man, the inspiring hero who, avoiding the constraints and exploiting the freedom of the system, uses his skill, charm, and luck to rise above the average.

Certainly the present system *allows* taking risks in ways that others may not. As such, it allows technical creativity as well as spectacular economic success. However, one must always remember that the system allows stupid and dangerous risks just as much as brilliant risks: failure is as easy as success. One rightly measures some of the value of a system by its successes, but one must also evaluate it by its average and its failures. I submit that the solo fee-for-service system of practice, as reflected in the level of performance of average practitioners, counteracts many of the virtues of the present system of medical education and will continue to do so regardless of any change one may make in medical education. I suggest that effective changes in average physician performance can be brought about more by modifying the social structure of practice than by changing the present education of medical students.

Designing Medical Practice: A Preliminary Illustration

The purpose of this chapter is not primarily to outline my critical views on the organization of medical care, for I shall save them for the end of this book. Instead, I am anticipating my later discussion to illustrate the way the idea of social structure may be used to understand medical care better and to indicate how distinctively different it is from ideas more closely connected with the common-sense individualism characteristic of medical thinking. As part of that illustration, it seems useful to indicate in a general way how one might modify the structure of medical practice to improve the quality of care.

The central problem is the quality of the performance of the practitioner. His performance must conform to the current technical standards of the academic leaders of his profession, maintain a decent and humane relationship with his patients, and give him enough satisfaction to make his work worth doing. To the extent to which his practice is such that (1) only his patients know how he does his work, (2) only his patients reward him for his work, and (3) his patients have other ready alternatives to his care, he may be expected to be pleasing to his patients but not especially up-to-date or careful by current medical standards. The problem is to keep him in some way accountable to and dependent upon his *patients'* approval while his work is at the same time observed and stimulated by *colleagues* oriented to keeping up with current technical standards.

If we look at these two conditions closely, we see that conventional practice arrangements are not directly relevant to them. There is a tendency to be dogmatic about one arrangement over another for doctrinaire reasons. Some people emphasize for its own sake the value of independent versus cooperative arrangements in the case of solo versus group practice. Others emphasize group practice because it has the ideological overtones of Community. Group practice, which is emphasized by the avant garde of medical policy makers and which I shall discuss in more detail later on, can easily be indifferent to both patients and technical standards and its cost need not be lower than that of solo practice. Careful attention to the *structural* implications of various arrangements can show us many alternatives, including the use of solo practice as a foundation for organization.

Ignoring economic issues, one can conceive of maintaining solo practice as it now exists, in individual offices well distributed throughout local neighborhoods and communities. It could even be maintained on an insured fee-for-service foundation, guarding against charges for an excessive number of services by statistical analysis of a type already in use in some Blue Shield plans. Poor technical practice can be guarded against by periodic review of a sample of medical records and physical examination of a sample of patients. The physician's desire to keep up and to conform to current standards can be stimulated by drawing him into consultative interaction with the arbiters of good practice—not leaving him with colleagues with similar problems and therefore similar standards, as is now the case.

This, of course, is only one possibility, sketched out so briefly here only to indicate that the simple shibboleths current in medical policy making confuse historical and ideological with analytical variables. What is essential to any arrangement is the preservation of enough leverage for the patient to avoid what Richard Titmuss called professional syndicalism[4] and to prevent the solidification of comfortable, like-minded colleagues into exclusive groups. It is a problem of engineering a judicious set of cross-pressures into the structure of practice which will motivate the practitioner to be, or to remain, what he was trained to be. And it is a problem that cannot be addressed persuasively at this stage of my exposition without exploration of the critical structural variables of medical care.

The Profession as an Element of Social Structure

It is my thesis that the most important single element in the social structure of medical care is the medical profession itself. Consonant with the structural approach I have discussed in this chapter, I shall not treat the profession as a collection of individuals with special knowledge and ethical orientations. Rather, I shall discuss the profession as an occupation with a special form of organization, a special form of legal "powers" analogous to that of bureaucratic officials, and a special position of dominance in the set of occupations that provide health care. Taken together, these structural characteristics of the profession have far more influence on the nature of medical care in the United States than either the good intentions and skills of individual members of the profession or the economic and administrative arrangements that are usually the focus of attempts at reform. In the next three chapters I will analyze them in some detail, beginning with a general examination of medicine as a profession.

NOTES

1. Phillip Rieff, *Freud, Mind of the Moralist* (Garden City, N. Y.: Doubleday, 1961), pp. 361 ff.
2. For elaboration of some of the succeeding remarks, see Eliot Freidson, *Patients' Views of Medical Practice* (New York: Russell Sage Foundation, 1961), Part 3. See also Eliot Freidson, *Profession of Medicine* (New York: Dodd-Mead, 1970), Chapter 5.
3. See O. L. Peterson et al., "An Analytical Study of North Carolina General Practice," *Journal of Medical Education*, 31 (December 1956), Part 2. See also Kenneth F. Clute, *The*

General Practitioner (Toronto, Ont.: University of Toronto Press, 1963).

4. Richard Titmuss, *Essays on "The Welfare State"* (London: Allen and Unwin, 1958), pp. 200–202.

Part 2

THE POSITION OF THE PROFESSION IN THE MEDICAL CARE STRUCTURE

3

The Profession—An Overview

The physician is the most prominent among members of the generally recognized professions. He is seen by the public as possessing a higher standard than any other professional and by the sociologist as the virtual prototype of his kind. While it would be a great mistake to confound what is peculiar to medicine with what is characteristic of professions in general, the study of physicians does offer the sociologist the opportunity to test both the truth and the utility of various orientations toward the concept of a profession.

One orientation sees a profession as an aggregate of people finding identity in sharing values and skills absorbed during a course of intensive training through which they all have passed. In this view the professional is primarily a particular kind of person; one determines whether or not an individual "is" a professional by determining whether or not he has internalized certain given professional values. One explains a "bad" professional by reference to his inferior education, his defective character, or similar variables. In short, one explains the behavior of members of a profession by reference to individual attributes and experiences bearing on conformity to a given set of norms.

Another orientation sees the profession as a group of workers joined together on the most general level by virtue of sharing a particular position in society and by common participation in a given division of labor. More specifically, the behavior of the profession is interpreted by referring to the way in which its work life is organized and to the pressures toward conformity or deviance implicit in that organization. Here the general assumption is that one defines a professional by his status, regardless of the norms to which he subscribes, and explains his behavior by referring to the work structure in which he participates.

One difficulty in assessing the virtues of each of these orientations is the fact that there have been few attempts to test them by sustained and detailed analysis of a single profession. Also, there has been little of the comprehensive comparative analysis that must be the ultimate goal of the sociology of medicine. Furthermore, because one of the marked characteristics of established professions is their relative freedom from lay intervention, from the conventional discipline exercised by industrial employers, and from the detailed directives of crafts unions, both organization and structure have been difficult to perceive. Professional organization is usually taken to be synonymous with the formal professional association, and the actual organization of work or practice has gone largely unnoticed.

This chapter, by attempting analysis of the medical profession and by focusing particularly on the way the performance of medical work is controlled, will try to clarify both the sociological characteristics of the medical profession and some of the issues germane to the sociology of the professions.[1] Because of the paucity of systematic empirical studies from other countries, it is regrettably necessary to run the risk of parochialism and concentrate on medicine in the United States.

Medicine and the State

The foundation on which the analysis of a profession must be based is its relationship to the ultimate source of power and authority in modern society—the state. In the case of medicine, much, though by no means all, of the profession's strength is based on legally supported monopoly over practice.[2] This monopoly operates through a system of licensing that bears on the privilege to hospitalize patients and the right to prescribe drugs and order laboratory procedures that are otherwise virtually inaccessible. It is the state that grants this monopoly, the exact form of which varies widely throughout the world.

In the United States the profession, through its private associations, has very largely been given the right to determine how political and legal power bearing on medicine shall be exercised.[3] In such countries as Great Britain, where the state has set up a national health system, representatives of the independent and private professional associations sit on both policy making and administrative boards and negotiate with the state on various issues influencing practice.[4] In the national health system of the Soviet Union there are no really private or independent representatives of the profession who can negotiate with the state, although advisory and administrative councils do include physicians.[5]

Clearly, the economic and political autonomy of the medical profession varies from country to country. What seems invariant, however, is its technological or scientific autonomy, for everywhere the profession appears to be left fairly free to develop its special area of knowledge and to determine what are "scientifically acceptable" practices.

In national state health systems, although laymen do serve in policy making and administrative positions, physicians tend to be administrative heads of practicing units and to be responsible for the determination of technical standards of equipment, procedures, and performance. Thus, while the profession may not everywhere be free to control the *terms* of its work, it is free to control the *content* of its work. Similarly, it is free to control the technical instruction of its recruits.

Medical Training

Quite as much as most sociologists, the medical profession considers medical education to be the major single factor determining the performance of the practicing professional. By the content of his education the student is "socialized" to become a physician. The assumption is that in the course of such an education a new kind of person is created. Medical education in the United States is perhaps unparalleled by any other conventional professional training in its duration, its detail, and its rigidity. Medical school lasts four years after undergraduate college, followed by a fifth year of supervised practice in an accredited teaching hospital (the internship), and even more years for those seeking certification as specialists. It would seem reasonable to think that such intensive exposure in fact molds the student into a particular kind of person. The Columbia University study of medical education[6] sought to demonstrate that the student, in the course of his training, develops a conception of himself as a doctor, absorbs the knowledge he needs to be secure enough to deal with patients without too much anxiety, and attains the capacity to cope with basic uncertainty in clinical practice.

Nonetheless, the students' perspective on their educational experience differs from that of their instructors. Indeed, one may expect some conflict between students and faculty by the very nature of their different roles. The unique contribution of the University of Kansas study[7] was its demonstration of the clash of perspectives in medical school and its finding that the differences in orientation leading to "restriction of production" are not limited to industrial organizations. The consequences of these findings for the educational process were followed up in some detail. But the study also emphasized that the existence of this clash of orientations did not mean that the performance of students and the demands of faculty had nothing in common. It was discovered that two dominant values held by the faculty were adopted by the students and used by them to guide their learning experience and select their careers. These were the values of medical responsibility and clinical experience.[8]

The value of medical responsibility refers to the traditional ideals of medicine, according to which the physician holds the life of a patient in his hands. It is the personal responsibility held by the physician working directly with a patient that requires him to take the blame for bad results. In the Kansas study it was found that this value was impressed on the student by frequent faculty lectures about the way mistakes of omission or commission endanger the patient's life. Furthermore, faculty members frequently asked students how they would handle an emergency so as to avoid serious consequences to the patient. The value was also featured in the organization of the training hospital, where the hierarchy of medical staff was ordered by differential access to medical responsibility, so that the unlicensed student was restricted to routine work having little relationship to life-or-death issues and the highest status person was free to carry out the most complicated and dangerous procedures.

Clinical experience refers to first-hand contact with patients and disease. Such contact is the ultimate justification for deciding to use one procedure for a treatment rather than another, and the experience so gained is valued because it provides a basis for therapeutic choice that is believed to be superior not only to the abstract considerations posed in textbooks but even to general, scientifically verified knowledge. It was observed in the course of the Kansas study that argument from experience was unanswerable except by the same type of argument from someone with greater experience.

These two values, Becker and his colleagues argued, order the choices the student makes from the range of experience offered by the medical school. These choices limit and direct his efforts in ways not anticipated or approved by the faculty. One of the student's most difficult problems is to select from the enormous mass of facts presented to him the information he is really to learn, for he cannot learn it all. The idea of clinical experience, it was suggested, guides his selection of facts and information and leads him to discount basic science and focus on classes in which instructors give practical information not found in books—information that adds to his store of vicarious experience. By the same token, he struggles for personal clinical experience in his training, avoiding routines he has already mastered. Similarly, he seeks tasks in which medical responsibility is apparent—reflecting some risk of danger—and avoids those in which it is not. Finally, he responds positively to some patients as cases presenting him with valued responsibility and experience and negatively to others as cases that take up a great deal of time without any valuable recompense.[9]

The evidence seemed to show that choice of career also hinges on how far specialties provide the opportunity for medical responsibility and clinical experience. Thus, a desirable specialty is one which offers a wide variety of experience and in which responsibility is symbolized by the possibility of killing or disabling patients in the course of making a mistake. Internal medicine, general surgery, and pediatrics are therefore the most popular specialties, although the potentially "mechanical" character of surgery and the necessity of liking to work with children in pediatrics qualify their desirability for some students. At the other extreme specialties like dermatology and allergy are unpopular because they are thought to involve little danger (and therefore little responsibility) or little variety.[10] National surveys of medical students in the United States have accumulated a fair amount of data on specialty choice, most of which are compatible with this interpretation of the values underlying the choices of the majority of students. In the case of those choosing the less popular specialties—the best investigated of which is public health[11]—specification of more detailed patterns of values is, of course, necessary.

Empirical Types of Practice

Unmentioned in the course of discussion of medical training is one element of great relevance to performance: the technical knowledge and skill learned by the student. Here it is necessary to say only that the student does in fact gain command over a great deal of knowledge and skill; what we must dwell on is the fact that this knowledge and skill is not necessarily retained or used after graduation from medical school. While in a modern industrial country like the United States all physicians share the same basic technical education, they do not all practice in the same way. In the few systematic studies of medical practice that have been made, it was found that the association between medical education and subsequent performance was at best very weak. While the available evidence is scanty and poor, it points to variation in the organization of practice—that is, in the organized setting in which the professional works—as a more important influence than medical education on variation in performance.[12] The analysis of work organization or practice is a critical problem for the sociology of professions.

The central issue in the analysis of work is control of performance. This issue constitutes a special problem for the analysis of professional work because professions, unlike other occupations, have successfully gained freedom from control by outsiders. Indeed, a profession is said to control its own performance. This is a rather unusual arrangement, worth understanding both for itself, as one type of control, and in its bearing on how, in our complex world, freedom and autonomy can be joined with responsibility. Let us examine the various organized practices in which medical work takes place to see how control over performance can be exercised.

One type of practice frequently held up as the ideal by professionals is that in which the individual is an entrepreneur, free to do what his own conscience and knowledge dictate. This is so-called solo practice. While pure forms of solo practice are quite rare (invoking it as a norm reflects the individualistic ideology of the profession more than it reflects reality), we might ask what conditions must be met to assure that individuals practicing entirely on their own conform to professional standards. Assurance of adequate performance on the part of solo practitioners seems to require exceedingly careful recruitment policies and extraordinarily effective educational procedures. In essence, the practitioner must be able to resist all temptations to ethical or technical lapses by virtue of his inner resources alone, resources which must also motivate him to continue to keep up to date. In solo practice the burden of control rests solely on individual motivation and capacity.

Much more common than solo practice in the United States today is practice involving a loose network of interdependent practitioners who refer cases to one another—an informal organization that has been described as a "colleague network."[13] Backed by a stable clientele relatively loyal to them, the practitioners in such a network control access to that clientele and thus access to work on the part of new, young practitioners. In the rather well-organized case he studied, Hall showed how an "inner fraternity" of practitioners controlled access to practice settings and desirable patients and how, through the mechanism of sponsorship, newcomers were obliged both to take minor tasks and to turn to their sponsors for consultation. While it may be doubted that professional services in large cities can be wholly dominated by any single informal fraternity, the sociometric studies of Coleman and his colleagues[14] suggest that there are systematic and persistent patterns of interrelationships among practitioners even in so loosely organized a system as exists in the United States. These patterns of interaction suggest two of the most important prerequisites for control of the practitioner's performance by colleagues rather than by clients: by referring patients to one another, each practitioner has the opportunity to *observe* some of the others' performance; by being economically and technically interdependent, each practitioner has some leverage to *influence* the others' performance.

Finally, one may mention the less primitive structures of practice that are characteristic of some European countries and are represented in the United States by large group practices and university clinics. These are essentially bureaucratic organizations, although the variations in actual administrative detail are countless. We may point to one logically distinct type of bureaucracy that has received some theoretical attention in the literature because of its systematic deviation from the classical rational–legal model of bureaucracy. It has been called *professional* bureaucracy and has been characterized as a form of organization in which the hierarchy of professional practitioners is set apart from the hierarchy of the administration itself, or (as in many European countries), a form of organization in which all important positions of organizational authority are filled by professionals. In both cases, professional work is free from the exercise of the authority of nonprofessionals even though the working professionals are technically subordinates in a bureaucratic system and lack the freedom of the entrepreneur.[15] The exact theoretical importance of such a logical construct and the degree to which it mirrors enough of reality to be useful are by no means clear, but by pointing to the bureaucratic elements of organization it does indicate that here, more than in other forms of practice, physicians are in a position of interdependence that implies opportunities to observe and to exercise influence over one another's performance. Of all types of practice reviewed, the bureaucratic type provides the best opportunity for professional self-regulation. Indeed, this is the type exemplified by high-prestige academic institutions in the United States and elsewhere.

Analytical Types of Practice

Thus far it has been suggested that there is a range of practice organizations, from purely individual practice to bureaucratically organized practice. To understand how colleagues or clients may gain access to observe and influence performance, it is useful to distinguish those features of practice that determine both the source and the content of control. In this way it becomes possible to analyze the differential significance in the division of labor of various forms of specialization. The lay client's perspective on the service he seeks differs from that of the colleague group of professionals; this may be taken as axiomatic. Let us therefore distinguish practices by the degree to which they are amenable to lay or colleague control. It is clear that two types of medical practice form the logical extremes of the medical division of labor. At one extreme is practice wholly dependent on lay choice for its existence; it may be called *client-dependent* practice. Such a practice survives by using its own resources to attract and satisfy a lay clientele. Since the client uses lay standards in deciding that he needs professional services and in evaluating the services he gets, the practice must conform to lay standards in order to be patronized. Furthermore, when wholly dependent on client choice, the practice cannot be observed by colleagues, nor is its survival dependent on their cooperation. In consequence, all the pressure on the practice is toward conforming to lay rather than professional standards. At the other extreme is *colleague-dependent* practice. It does not attract its own lay clientele but rather obtains clients through the referrals of other colleagues. Thus, in order to survive it must honor the prejudices of colleagues, and so is likely to conform more to professional than to lay standards.

How closely do actual practices conform to these logical types? The logical extreme of client-dependent practice does not seem fully applicable to any professional practice, although the "independent" solo neighborhood or village general practitioner comes close to it. Also close are specialists who must attract a clientele directly and do not have to make everyday use of hospital facilities—for example, particularly in urban areas, some internists, pediatricians, ophthalmologists, and gynecologists. In these instances lay standards may be expected to have some force. Empirical examples of the logical extreme of colleague-dependent practices are easier to find in modern medicine. Specialists like pathologists and radiologists, for instance. are almost completely dependent upon colleague referrals and therefore have little need for such client-oriented techniques as a good bedside manner. Here we should expect considerably greater pressure to honor colleague rather than lay or patient standards.

This typology is based on the division of labor within the profession and is therefore applicable to analysis of the control of performance of individual practitioners in any kind of organized practice, from solo to bureaucratic. It might be pointed out, however, that in bureaucratically organized practice it is frequently the organization as a unit, not individual practitioners, which attracts a clientele, and all practitioners in the organization are therefore dependent on it for their work. Insofar as the organization is of the "professional" type just discussed, this means that dependence on it is actually dependence on the colleagues running it. Encouragement to meet professional standards of performance will therefore be considerably stronger than encouragement to meet lay standards. And insofar as work is at once more visible and amenable to control in such an organization than in less well-organized forms of practice, it is here that we should expect to find the highest professional standards. Indeed, it is the general opinion of teachers of medicine in the United States, Great Britain, and elsewhere that this is the case, although adequate evidence to test this opinion has not yet been gathered.

All else being equal, then, we may hypothesize that colleague-dependent practices, in which the physician's performance is observable to colleagues and his work dependent on colleagues, will also be most likely to conform to professional standards. Insofar as bureaucratic practice is colleague-dependent, the same conclusion may be drawn for it. But this conclusion masks several assumptions the truth of which is not self-evident: first, that colleagues will exert control over performance; second, that the mechanisms of control used by colleagues are effective; third, that standards are homogeneous throughout the profession. The remainder of this chapter will explore these assumptions.

Professional Regulation

Variation in the organization of medical practice bears on such necessary conditions for the exercise of professional regulation as the observability of performance to colleagues and the structural vulnerability of the practitioner to control by colleagues. However, while observability and dependence are necessary conditions for the effective exercise of supervision, they are not sufficient. What is needed in addition is willingness to exercise supervision and exert effective influence over performance. What slender evidence there is suggests that rather less influence over performance is exercised than the organization of practice actually allows, and that the little regulation that does exist has properties that establish and maintain organized differences in performance standards.

The basic property of the system of control that seems to exist in the United States is its reliance upon what Carr-Saunders and Wilson call the "boycott"—that is, the refusal by individual practitioners to enter into a referral or collaborative relationship with those of whom they do not approve.[16] This device does not control the boycotted person's behavior so much as it pushes him outside the boundaries of observability and influence, to practice as he wishes in the company of those with similar standards. There seems to be a certain reluctance to exert active influence over another's performance—a reluctance that results in avoiding him rather than in seeking to change his practices.

There is, unfortunately, little systematically collected empirical information bearing on the process of supervision and control among physicians. A study by Freidson and Rhea[17] of a large academically oriented group practice in the United States indicated that while performance was visible along the axes dictated by the interdependence of specialties within the over-all division of labor, each practitioner tended to keep his complaints about others to himself, so that what he could observe of others' performance in the division of labor was not transmitted to other colleagues. Since bits of information were scattered piecemeal through the colleague group, no really organized control of performance could be initiated unless a man behaved so outrageously as to personally offend everyone. Furthermore, attempts at control were largely individual and hortatory, and there were no control devices intermediate between remonstrance and outright ejection from the organization (the latter being the structural equivalent of the boycott). While the physicians studied were aware of the looseness of supervision and control in this ostensibly well-organized practice, they were inclined to feel it adequate and appropriate for ordinary circumstances.

Another American study is particularly instructive because it was done in a setting into which supervision was built.[18] There were clear bureaucratic as well as professional supervisory responsibilities allocated through hierarchical ranks. The superior physician in the hierarchy had the right and perhaps even the obligation to review case records and evaluate case management. Furthermore, he had the right to give advice to subordinates about the way a case should be handled, even when advice was not solicited. However, even though the supervisor was officially responsible for the care given to patients in his unit and therefore had the formal right to order that certain procedures be followed for a case, he very rarely gave such orders. Instead, he gave advice, which incurred no obligation to obedience. The only obligation the subordinate had was to consider the advice in the light of his personal experience with and responsibility for the case. So long as he could justify his management of the case by reference to medical knowledge and his clinical experience, and so long as it was he who took personal responsibility for the outcome, he could reject the advice of his superior. In short, even here, where supervisory inspection of performance was routine, the exercise of control over performance was quite loose and permissive. If this is so in hierarchically organized practice settings, it should be even more the case in the informal, small-scale community practices that are far more common in medicine. Thus, we may say that the medical profession, which has gained freedom from regulation by others, regulates itself in ways whose effectiveness is not self-evident. The analytical problem here is to understand what contributes to shaping this peculiar process of regulation and to point out its structural consequences.

Professional Values

Obviously, when a social structure *permits* certain kinds of behavior but that behavior does not occur, we must explore the situation further to explain why it does not. Our first question might be why, in such a loose system, the physician does not routinely abuse his privilege. Here, the internalization of general professional values postulated by Parsons[19] seems a plausible explanation. Parsons defines the professional as someone who is supposed to be recruited and licensed on the basis of his technical competence rather than his ascribed social characteristics, to use generally accepted rather than particularistic scientific standards in his work, to restrict his work activity to areas in which he is technically competent, to avoid emotional involvement and to cultivate objectivity in his work, and to put his client's interests before his own. These normative expectations are intended by Parsons to apply to all professions, not only to medicine, since he treats the medical practitioner as the archetype of the professional. But it may be objected that the same expectations are applicable to all technical service occupations, not only to professions. Plumbers too are supposed to be recruited and licensed on the basis of achievement, to employ universalistic standards in their work, to be functionally specific and affectively neutral. And while plumbers are expected to make enough money from their work to gain a decent income (just as are physicians), they are not expected to do this by cheating the customer. Thus, such values constitute only the most general foundation of conscientiousness in occupational practice.

Our second question, however, may be more specific to the medical profession. Why, if it so conscientious, does it not exercise more regulation over its members' performance? Such an extraordinarily loose regulatory structure has been explained by Carr-Saunders and Wilson[20] and by Parsons[21] by reference to the character of professional work. Instead of a set routine, medicine requires the exercise of complex judgment; instead of caution, the taking of risks. Therefore, regulation can only be loose. But of all the old established professions medicine is the one most based on fairly precise and detailed scientific knowledge. Indeed, the practice of medicine involves considerably less uncertainty than many other technical occupations. As the use of the doctrine of *res ipsa loquitur* in American courts implies, there are some very clear rights and wrongs in medicine, even if there are also some uncertainties, and these rights and wrongs have not brought forth any formal regulatory mechanisms from the profession as such (as opposed to concrete organizations like teaching hospitals, in which regulatory mechanisms do exist). Without denying that there is a degree of uncertainty, we must conclude that the precision possible in much of modern medicine and the trivial routine of much of everyday medical practice call into question the adequacy of explaining the peculiarly loose structure of controls to be found in the profession by reference to the character of its work. However, it may be that the peculiar nature of the work of the practicing professional encourages a characteristic *sense* of uncertainty that reflects considerably more special values than those described by Parsons.

One such value is that of independence or autonomy, which is significant for physicians in countries as different as Finland and the United States. Insofar as this value refers to social and economic independence, it reflects the entrepreneurial and individualistic ideology of the bourgeoisie, who are the prime source from which physicians are recruited in virtually all industrial countries. Insofar as the value refers to technical or professional independence—that is, the freedom to practice one's craft without interference, advice, or regulation by others—it seems more closely related to a state of mind encouraged by the character of professional work.

The aim of the practitioner is not knowledge but action, and while successful action is the aim, the tendency is to assume that any action at all is better than none. Furthermore, to take action requires faith in oneself and even a will to believe in whatever one does instead of maintaining a skeptical detachment. Dealing with individual and concrete cases, the practitioner is inclined to emphasize indeterminacy rather than lawful regularity and to be radically pragmatic, relying more on the results he associates with his own actions than on theory. These seem to be the orientations that contribute to the emphasis on clinical experience mentioned earlier in connection with medical education.

Given that the work of the medical practitioner is with individuals and that it is believed to be based on individual clinical experience, it follows that responsibility for the work can be perceived only as individual and personal. In assuring that responsibility, the practitioner does gain gratitude for success, but he also risks reproach for failure. Given the risk of blame, he displays a certain sensitivity and defensiveness in the face of any outsider's evaluation of his performance. This defensiveness is manifested in imputing more uncertainty to the work than in fact exists and in insisting on using his own personal, clinical experience as the ultimate criterion for evaluating his own performance. Thus, collective responsibility for regulation is diminished and the inclination to rely on individual responsibility and personal experience is augmented.

These, of course, are merely suggestions of the complex task that has still to be done in picking out and interrelating strands of what might be called the ideology of the practicing professional. Instead of dwelling on values of such generality that they have doubtful analytical utility for understanding the quality of professional self-regulation, sociologists should determine the specific values attached to different types of professional work. Such an approach would supply one of the critical elements for an adequate explanation of the peculiarities of professional organization.

Informal Organization of the Profession

Even without detailed information it seems possible to suggest that the notion of informal organization serves as a vital link between the formal structure given to the American medical profession by the national, state, and county medical associations, and professional performance in the concrete setting of medical practice. By focusing on the characteristic way in which practitioners assert control over one another's performance, one can delineate the relation of one local practice to another and the loose groupings of practices that both carve up a community and extend outside its boundaries. When these informal groupings and the mechanisms of control they express are seen to be intertwined with the formal structure of the profession as a whole, much more of the character of the profession can be understood than by reference to formal associations and codes alone.

Recalling that ordinarily the ultimate mechanism of control is the personal boycott, we can begin to indicate the informal structure of the profession by following the implications of the boycott's operation on the interrelations of practitioners. Let us assume that individual practitioners are free to select the work they will undertake and to choose the colleagues with whom they will work in the division of labor. In this situation, control of professional standards is exercised largely by willingness to work with one man and to exclude another. But since exclusion as such neither changes a man nor prevents him from working, one may assume that he will eventually find a circle whose standards are such that he is not excluded.

There is thus a tendency for the control process to develop a stable set of colleague networks or fraternities. Each network, by the nature of its creation, is fairly homogeneous within itself. Its members share about the same professional standards, participate in one another's work, and participate in, if not dominate, the particular organizations and practices in which they work. But while each colleague network is likely to be fairly homogeneous, many differences are likely to exist *between* networks by virtue of the process of selection and rejection that differentiates them into separate networks. Thus there is not only likely to be little interaction between many contiguous networks but also marked differences in technical and normative standards and in the practices and institutions in which the members of each network participate.

In a structure of this nature there is comparatively little opportunity for those in one network to be very much aware of the existence of other standards, and even when awareness may exist, there is little leverage by which one network could influence another because each has severed connections with the other and is independent of the other. Since it is a segregating process that leads to and maintains such networks, and since the individual's behavior is less regulated by such a process than classified and assigned to a self-maintaining collectivity of like people, we can see how within a single profession, even one quite free of lay interference, organized variations in professional performance can occur. While there are certainly social links between adjacent fraternities in the form of practitioners with connections in both, it does not seem to require a very large city to find individual practitioners who know nothing about one another.

The characteristic control mechanism of professional regulation, then, paradoxically operates to place offenders beyond the control of those who disapprove of their performance. Moreover, the informal organization in internally homogeneous colleague networks segregated from interaction with each other sustains, if not reinforces, the differences in standards among networks. Apart from civil suit, which is a nonprofessional source of control over practice, and regulatory devices established in the limited milieu of teaching hospitals, all that is left to concerned members of the profession in the United States is exhortation and, it is hoped, instruction by means of articles in professional journals that may or may not be read and that, if read, may or may not influence behavior.

What has been suggested, in short, is that the disjunctive process of social control characterizing the concrete, everyday practice of American physicians creates an informal structure of relatively segregated, small circles of practitioners, the extremes of which are so isolated from each other that the conditions necessary for mutual influence on behavior are missing. Furthermore, the mechanism of control that produces and sustains the situation is no aberration—rather, it is characteristic of the profession, an outcome of its organization and of the way it sees itself and its work. The consequence is that a single profession can contain within itself, and even encourage, markedly different ethical and technical standards of performance, performance limited in a very superficial way by the minimal standards imposed by selective recruiting, a basic core of training required for licensing, and the writings of the leaders of the medical profession.

Tasks of Analysis

The problems of analysis described in this chapter are not unique to the sociology of medicine but affect the sociology of professions in general. If they can be solved for medicine, we will have taken a long step toward solving them for all professions. The central problem here, as in the study of society in general, is social control. The problem is particularly important for the professions because by definition they are free of the controls common to most occupations. In addressing the problem of control, it was necessary to assess the roles of the state and politico–legal institutions, the manifest and latent functions of professional education, the organization of work, and the norms or values that bear on the exercise of social control in work. The outcome of that analysis was the suggestion that a fragmented structure underlies the serene façade of unity and homogeneity implied by the notion of a single profession joined by common values and a community of identity.

To extend, correct, and refine such a trial analysis of the organization of medical work is one of the prime tasks of a sociology of medicine. In the course of extending it, one would be led quite naturally into a more detailed examination of another major problem of analysis, the client–practitioner relationship. This problem too might be seen as one of control. The practitioner wants the client to seek him out for professionally appropriate reasons, without visiting quacks and without untoward delay. He wants the client to accept his recommendations and follow them scrupulously. In seeking compliance on the part of his client, the professional cannot always rely on his influence as an expert. The character of this influence and of practitioner–client interaction has barely been explored in other than psychological terms and poses a challenge both to the taxonomy of types of social influence and to the conceptualization of social interaction. We will examine it more closely in the following chapter.

NOTES

1. This chapter is a partial summary of Parts I and II of my *Profession of Medicine* (New York: Dodd-Mead, 1970).
2. See Henry E. Sigerist, "The History of Medical Licensure," in Henry E. Sigerist, *On the Sociology of Medicine*, M. I. Roemer, ed. (New York: MD Publications, 1960).
3. A bit old now but still the essential reference is David R. Hyde et al., "The American Medical Association: Power, Purpose and Politics in Organized Medicine," *Yale Law Journal*, 60 (1954), 938–1022.
4. For a good discussion of the English scene, see Rosemary Stevens, *Medical Practice in Modern England* (New Haven, Conn.: Yale University Press, 1966).
5. For essential information on the Soviet system see Mark G. Field, *Soviet Socialized Medicine: An Introduction* (New York: The Free Press, 1967).
6. Robert K. Merton et al., eds., *The Student Physician* (Cambridge, Mass.: Harvard University Press, 1957).
7. Howard S. Becker et al., *Boys in White* (Chicago: University of Chicago Press, 1961).
8. *Ibid.*, Chapters 12 and 13.
9. *Ibid.*, Chapters 14 and 16.
10. *Ibid.*, Chapter 20.
11. Robert E. Coker, Jr., et al., "Medical Careers in Public Health," *Milbank Memorial Fund Quarterly*, 44 (1966), 143–258.

12. See Freidson, *Profession of Medicine*, Chapter 5.

13. Oswald Hall, "The Informal Organization of the Medical Profession," *Canadian Journal of Economics and Political Science*, 12 (1946), 30–44.

14. James A. Coleman et al., *Medical Innovation: A Diffusion Study* (Indianapolis, Ind.: Bobbs-Merrill, 1966).

15. See Gloria V. Engel, "The Effect of Bureaucracy on the Professional Autonomy of the Physician," *Journal of Health and Social Behavior*, 10 (1969), 30–41, and W. Richard Scott, "Reactions to Supervision in a Heteronomous Professional Organization," *Administrative Science Quarterly*, 10 (1965), 65–81.

16. A. M. Carr-Saunders and P. A. Wilson, *The Professions* (Cambridge: Oxford University Press, 1933), p. 403, and see also Hyde et al., "American Medical Association."

17. Eliot Freidson and Buford Rhea, "Processes of Control in a Company of Equals," *Social Problems*, 11 (1963), 119–131, and Eliot Freidson and Buford Rhea, "Knowledge and Judgment in Professional Evaluations," *Administrative Science Quarterly*, 10 (1965), 107–124.

18. Mary E. W. Goss, "Influence and Authority among Physicians in an Outpatient Clinic," *American Sociological Review*, 26 (1961), 39–50, and Mary E. W. Goss, "Patterns of Bureaucracy among Hospital Staff Physicians," in Eliot Freidson, ed., *The Hospital in Modern Society* (New York: The Free Press, 1963), pp. 170–194.

19. Talcott Parsons, *The Social System* (Glencoe, Ill.: The Free Press, 1951), Chapter 10.

20. Carr-Saunders and Wilson, *The Professions*, pp. 399–400.

21. Parsons, *Social System*, pp. 470–471.

4

The Structural Solution to the Problem of Professional Authority

It is my thesis that the relation of the physician to his clientele is inherently problematic. Indeed, the relation of any service occupation to its clientele is inherently problematic. Insofar as the occupation is truly an occupation rather than an occasional amateur activity, its members are bound to develop their own ways of looking at the problems its clientele brings. They are certain to typify and routinize those problems in ways with which those suffering from them for the first time are unlikely to concur, each sufferer being preoccupied with his uniqueness. As Hughes has pointed out, what is a critical emergency to the layman seeking help may be to the professional worker just another routine, common occurrence he has handled many times before.[1] While both consultant and client come together with the end in mind of managing the problem of the latter, each has a different perspective on the problem itself and on the means of managing it.

These differences in perspective are, as I have already

noted, a partial function of the occupational experience of the consultant which leads him to take a rather more routine view of the problem than the sufferer's. They are also, however, a function of the specialized knowledge implied both by occupational experience and by the formal training that professions, if not all occupations, provide their members. Indeed, one of the things that marks off professions from occupations is the professions' claim to schooling in knowledge of an especially esoteric, scientific, or abstract character that is markedly superior to the mere experience of suffering from the illness or of having attempted pragmatically to heal a procession of sufferers of the illness. Not merely difference in perspective enters into the client–professional relationship, therefore, but also difference in what is brought to that perspective. The professional, emphasizing theory or abstract knowledge, may be led to emphasize a treatment that seems to the patient to have no direct connection with the discomfort he feels. Now it is true that many recommendations contrary to common sense—such as that if the patient has a pain in his head he should put two white pills into his stomach—have become conventional enough to create no problems between consultant and client. But no matter how well educated the patient has been, he is bound to have his faith and confidence put to the test by some of the esoteric, superficially irrelevant recommendations that his physician will make. If the physician asserts esoteric knowledge, such events of strain cannot fail to occur by the nature of the case. The problem is how the physician manages the strain.

The Profession of Consultation

In analyzing the character of the profession's interaction with its clientele, it is necessary to make a distinction of some empirical and analytical importance between the kind of work medical practice is and the kind of work of similarly prestigious pursuits also often called "professional." Everett Hughes distinguished three occupational models: science, business, and profession. Of particular interest is his contrast between science and profession, a contrast that contradicts most usage in sociology and that has analytical consequences of some importance. He sees *science* as the pursuit of knowledge, its value hinging on convincing communication to colleagues. He sees *profession* as the giving of an esoteric service to a client who "has met a problem which he cannot himself handle."[2] Thus, the prime structural difference between profession and science is that one has a lay clientele and the other does not. From that difference flow consequences that negate the importance to analysis of what both have in common—the exercise of what is considered some esoteric knowledge, skill, or expertise.

In the case of science, similarly knowledgeable colleagues constitute the consumers of the practitioner's special skill. But in the profession, the consumers are lay clients. Thus, in a profession but not in a science, the worker may be on occasion "required in some measure to yield judgment of what is wanted to . . . amateurs who receive the services."[3] To protect both the professional and the client from the consequences of this, Hughes observes, the profession maintains secrecy in its affairs and orders its practice through such formal institutions as state licensing. Science, on the other hand, requires full and honest reporting and relies on informal controls. "Secrecy and institutional sanctions thus arise in the profession as they do not in the pure science."[4]

From this conclusion, however, flows an as yet unemphasized point, namely, that the type of influence or authority exerted by the professional on his clients must be quite different from that exerted by the scientist on his colleagues—that professional and scientific "authority" are different even though profession and science are both characterized by special technical competence. Indeed, I shall argue that professional "authority" is a logically mixed or impure case, containing some of the elements of the authority of technical competence and some of the elements of the authority of legal or bureaucratic office.

Official and Expert Authority

In his commentary on Max Weber's delineation of bureaucratic administration, Talcott Parsons notes that Weber overlooked the logical (or "pure") distinction between the authority of office and the "authority" of knowledge or technical competence. In a strictly logical sense, the capacity of the officeholder to influence the behavior of others (that is, to exert authority) is a function of the office he holds, with no necessary relation to how much he may have to know to do his official job. "Thus, the treasurer of a corporation is empowered to sign checks disbursing large funds. There is no implication in the 'power' that he is a more competent signer of checks than the bank clerks or tellers who cash or deposit them for the recipient. Legal 'competence' is a question of 'powers' in this sense; technical competence is of a different order."[5]

The logical distinction is certainly clear, but it does not tell us how each kind of "authority" elicits obedience. We can understand how the authority of the officeholder works in that it frequently rests on his capacity to sanction his subordinates—to withhold or to grant monetary rewards, for example. Part and parcel of the office is legitimate access to such sanctions. But, logically distinct from that of the officeholder, the "authority" of technical competence has no clear sanctions at its disposal. How, therefore, does it move others to "obey"? Parsons seems to believe that the profession in general and the medical profession in particular exemplify the authority of technical competence. How does the professional move clients to "obey"? How does this differ from the way scientists move colleagues to accept their findings?

In each case, we can see the problem as one of persuasion. But if we recall Hughes's distinction between science and profession we see that the problem of persuasion is very different for each. In science, the practitioner deals with colleagues who share his premises and basic knowledge and who are inclined to accept his findings (that is, be influenced by him) when they conform to common rules of evidence and procedure. Authority here is based on persuasion grounded in a common universe of discourse, a shared set of paradigms.[6] By the nature of the case it is very different for the practicing professional, who must exert his authority over laymen. Unlike colleagues, lay clients do not necessarily share the professional's universe of discourse. Indeed, lay clients are by definition lacking in the educational or experiential prerequisites that would allow them to decide, on grounds shared with the professional, whether to accept any particular piece of professional advice. In this sense, the professional's grounds for persuading his clients to obey him are inherently problematic and the problem of professional authority therefore distinctly different from that of scientific authority.

The problem of professional authority is the same as the problem posed to all workers who give consultative services to laymen. Any expert whose work characteristically requires the cooperation of laymen is handicapped because laymen know neither the occupational rules of evidence nor the basic content of his skill. *What distinguishes the professional from all other consulting experts is his capacity to solve some of these problems of authority by formal, institutional means. His solution minimizes the role of persuasive evidence in his interaction with his clientele.* Thus, by virtue of his institutionalized solutions to the problem, the professional, even more than consulting experts in general, exercises a kind of authority that is markedly different from that of the scientist.[7]

Problems of Cultural and Educational Difference

Without such an institutional solution to the problem of conflict, I believe, medical work would be considerably more difficult than it is. The issue of perspective is insoluble, for while the physician can in some sense sympathize with the patient, he must maintain his detachment from the patient's responses or else lose his effectiveness by becoming merely a sympathetic friend. Some element of conflict is thus bound to occur as long as both client and consultant play their role properly, for the perspective of the client is such that he cannot really merely place himself in the consultant's hands as he is told to. The conflict surrounding differential knowledge, however, is one that many writers seem to feel can be minimized, if not absolutely eliminated, by changes in the behavior of either physician or patient. Let us look at the problem a bit more closely.

We might distinguish two types of difference in knowledge and belief. First, there is the difference to be found between, let us say, an American physician and an American patient. Let us assume that insofar as they are both acculturated Americans they share much the same values of health, conceptions of illness, and notions of the proper ways for patients and doctors to behave. The critical difference between them is essentially formal professional education and accumulated occupational experience. The better educated in medicine the patient is, the more like the doctor he will be. Second, however, there is the difference to be found between an American physician and, let us say, an Indian peasant. There the difference does not lie solely in the lack of formal education in medicine but in the very premises about the nature of health and illness, the etiquette of consultation, and the proper roles for patient and healer.

Let us for convenience call the first difference "educational" and the second "cultural" and ask how each may be resolved. The cultural difference is patently the most serious, for depending on whose point of view you take, the doctor or the patient will fail to conform to what the other would consider the most elementary rules governing consultation. The patient may be outraged that the physician asks him what his symptoms are rather than telling him what they are and what has caused them.[8] Or the physician may be outraged that the patient refuses to pay until he is satisfied with the efficacy of his treatment. So long as such cultural differences exist, physicians are unlikely to have much access to patients, for they will not be consulted regularly and matter-of-factly. And when he does come into contact with such patients, it is incumbent upon the physician who wishes to work to in some way understand his patients' culture sufficiently to be able to teach them something of his point of view and, where that is not possible, to modify his own behavior to conform with the patients' expectations rather than lose the patients.

Clearly, however, there are limits to the extent to which the physician can adjust to the culture of his patients, limits that are set by his own occupational integrity. It is true that physicians are prone to be reluctant to change their approach in ways that have nothing to do with the professional quality of their treatment, but their knowledge and technique in themselves set limits past which they cannot go without ceasing to be physicians. While the physician anxious to please can offer a money-back guarantee like any reputable village healer without damaging his medical technique, he cannot substitute a poultice of cow dung for an injection of antibiotic in the treatment of a bacterial infection. When his patients are markedly different from him, he cannot satisfy them without giving up his profession. Assuming that he remains a physician, this means that where there are cultural differences between patient and profession, there is also conflict that can only partially be reduced by sympathy, understanding, and good will, and by-passed by mutual avoidance; the profession must manage that conflict in some way if it is to be able to do its work.

Educational differences between patient and practitioner are rather less a problem than cultural differences, but they are a problem nonetheless. Essentially, the solution is seen to lie in "health education"—that is, in the patient's being taught enough about modern medicine to be able to approach his illness from the same perspective as the physician and to be sufficiently informed about the nature of illness that he will understand what the physician says and so be able to cooperate intelligently. There are, however, more problems connected with such health education than its advocates seem to recognize. These problems become apparent when we think of the characteristic interaction between the practitioner and the least educated. The least-educated client is exemplified by infants and animals in the absence of their owners. They cannot be counted on to seek help nor can they cooperate intelligently with the practitioner's attempts to cope with their problem. In compensation to the practitioner, they may be managed by simple means of physical restraint rather than by complex and time-consuming persuasion, but they obviously leave something to be desired as patients. In contrast, optimal cooperation might be expected from the best-educated client. But when we remember that the best-educated client is the practitioner himself in need of consultation, we must acknowledge that such a client is notoriously troublesome; in the Soviet Union as well as in the United States the physician is a notoriously poor patient. The professional is a poor client precisely because he knows too much. Because he knows too much he cannot give up his own conception of his problem and its solution and submit to the authority of his consultant. Health education, then, solves some part of the problem of conflict and compliance but only at the expense of intensifying another part of the problem.

Professional Prestige

A more common solution to the problem lies in the socioeconomic position of the professional and the prestige of his profession. Though not often noted explicitly as a solution to the conflict of expectations, one does often hear references to the necessity of preserving the dignity of the profession and to the confidence instilled by a doctor who looks successful, drives a Cadillac, and dresses well.[9] In the face of such inspiring impressions, the patient may swallow his anxiety and restrain his demands, feeling that the physician is too important to be bothered by the trivial or that he is too busy to be expected to explain. Furthermore, the patient may grant deference to the physician because the physician is of an upper middle-class background and is a member of an old, honorable, and superlatively prestigious profession. The exercise of such deference is manifested in the exercise of a certain passivity and restraint on the part of the client; even if he feels a certain uneasiness at the physician's method or prescription, the client's uneasiness will remain muted, and the physician is likely to have the feeling that all goes smoothly.

The solution, however, may be more apparent than real. More than one writer has noted that where status differences between client and practitioner are so great as to require deference in interaction, the client may be so uncomfortable and fearful as to avoid consultation in the first place. Perhaps this is why James IV of Scotland, in the course of practicing medicine himself, paid a fee to his patients rather than vice versa: perhaps they would not have come in otherwise.[10] Furthermore, once in consultation, patients markedly lower in status than their physician can be so intimidated as to be reluctant to engage in the exchanges necessary for adequate diagnosis and prescription, and, by virtue of the restraints imposed by the necessity of deference, may subsequently evade contact with the professional.

Furthermore, we may note that while the very character of the distribution of status through the population is such that the upper middle-class practitioner will in most cases be treating his status subordinates, there are instances in which he treats superordinates. Under those circumstances it is the practitioner who is vulnerable. Superordinate patients tend to be rather more imperious and demanding and to assume that the practitioner exists for their convenience and as an instrument for their own therapeutic prejudices. Whereas in the instance of status superiority the physician dominates treatment at the risk of losing his patients, in the instance of status subordination the physician must allow the patients to dominate treatment at the risk of losing them.

Institutional Impurities in Professional Authority

Thus far I have pointed out the nature of the conflict to be found between physician and layman, and I have assessed the roles of cultural, educational, and status differences in resolving or increasing that conflict. These differences are involved in any relationship between consulting expert and client. What is special about the consulting profession in general and the physician in particular is the use of formal institutional solutions that make his authority as great if not greater than that of the official.

In order to work, the practicing expert must gain access to clientele. Such access is contingent on the client's having failed to solve a problem himself. When the suburban householder has taken apart a defective fixture and cannot restore it to work even as badly as before, or when the ailing soul has dosed himself only to feel worse than he felt originally, he is inclined to seek the aid of someone else. Since the expert will not be sought out unless others know of his existence, he must establish some kind of visibility through a public identity and be known to those most likely to need the services he offers. Given a public identity, the expert will thrive if he is able to obtain some assurance that people seeking the services he offers will be likely to seek them from him and not from just anyone pretending to his skill.

The professional solves the problem of access to a clientele in a manner that sets him apart from the general class "consulting expert." Characteristically, as Hughes pointed out, his public identity is institutionalized and he gains at least a quasi-monopoly over the right to do the work he does. The solution of the professional is to have himself designated as the expert in such a way as to exclude all other claimants, his designation being official and bureaucratic insofar as it is formally established by law. Thus, with slight exception, only the physician has the legal right to practice medicine, perform surgery, write prescriptions, and certify compensation claims and sick leaves. Insofar as the professional solution to gaining access to a clientele relies upon incumbency in such an official, licensed position, it may justifiably be called "bureaucratic" even though (like the notary public who has a private practice of "legal powers") it does not take place within a formal administrative organization as circumscribed as a bureau or corporation. Because of its official position the profession is better assured than the mere expert that the people seeking the services it offers will have to seek them from its members or not at all. Logically, the "powers" of office are crucial,[11] though as I shall note later, technical competence may be important in encouraging the public decision to establish the official position and lay down formal technical qualifications for its incumbents. Therefore, the prospective clientele of the profession, unlike that of the mere expert, is captive in a closed universe of practitioners established in an official position in society.

But this is not enough. Like an expert, the professional is handicapped in his exercise of authority because he cannot wield the sanctions normally attached to bureaucratic office or legal authority. The horse may be led to water by limiting the direction his paths take, but how may he be made to drink? Since the client is led to the expert by his own layman's view of his problem, there is a very good chance that the client will want something contrary to what the expert may feel is appropriate. The only real sanction the expert has over his client is the threat to withhold service, but if the service is not that which the layman wants anyway, the sanction is singularly hollow. What is characteristic of the profession's solution to this problem lies not only in its capture of exclusive control over the exercise of a particular skill but also in its capture of the exclusive right of access to goods and services the layman is likely to feel he needs to manage his own problem himself, independently of expert advice.

By becoming a gatekeeper to what is popularly valued, the professional gains the additional sanction of being able to make taking his advice a prerequisite for obtaining a good or service valued independently of his advice. Thus, the layman may feel he knows exactly what drug he needs, but nonetheless he must go to a physician for a prescription; one may be fully persuaded he knows what he needs to learn to be entitled to a degree or educational certificate, but he must nonetheless do what the teachers ask to get the grades and credits prerequisite to the certificate. In contrast, one need not go to an automobile mechanic to get the spare parts needed to fix one's automobile oneself (even though automobile manufacturers sometimes manage to require this).

The more strategic the accessories controlled by the profession, then, the stronger the sanctions supporting its authority. However, it is of critical importance to that authority that the layman not have even more powerful sanctions himself, for history is replete with instances in which weakly organized experts have been required to devote themselves to giving what powerful clients thought best rather than to giving them the measured fruits of expert opinion.[12] Of course, when this occurs, professional authority has collapsed, if indeed a profession can be said to exist at all. To buttress its members' authority against unmanageable pressure, the profession seeks to limit its number and to establish circumstances that prevent the clientele from organizing as a corporate body. When the number of its members is small in relation to demand and when the clientele is unorganized, individual practitioners are in a position to be able to refuse inappropriate client requests without courting economic or political ruin.

Outcomes of Institutionalization

All the devices I have mentioned thus far constitute ways of institutionalizing practice to limit and channel the behavior of the layman, bringing him into consultation with the professional under circumstances in which he has few alternatives for action. Influence is not exerted by adducing persuasive evidence that professional advice is valid and therefore worth obeying. Reliance is on the "legal" authority of institutionalized competence. Let us try to visualize more clearly the implications of such institutionalization by examining the alternative interactions it allows between client and practitioner. Let us remember that we are confronted by an occupation that has gained monopoly over the right to offer a given set of services, including a monopoly over access to some of the resources needed to manage a given set of problems related to the services. Furthermore, the members of the occupation are relatively few in number and its clientele is a large, unorganized aggregate of individuals, leaving little possibility for the exertion of lay pressure to compromise occupationally preferred standards. What are the practical alternatives for the interaction between practitioner and client, and what kind of influence is exercised in each case?

If the practitioner's advice or service does not conform

to the desires of the client, the client may merely withdraw from the situation when he realizes that he cannot get the practitioner to conform to his own desires. Here, no authority of any kind is exercised. But since he desires some resource which he can obtain only by at least temporarily accepting what the practitioner "suggests," the client may give in and do what the physician advises. Here conformity is obtained because of command over accessory resources by the practitioner rather than because the client recognizes or accepts the value of the practitioner's competence. In some cases, the practitioner's advice is accepted because it happens to correspond to what the client expects or desires, whether or not the grounds for the client's expectations are the same as those of the practitioner. That the practitioner is a professional or an expert may be wholly irrelevant, as may be the notion of authority itself; if this is the case, there has been a mere convergence of opinion. In still other cases, the client becomes persuaded in the course of his interaction with the practitioner that the latter's advice is in his best interest, whether or not it happens to conform with what he initially believed he needed. Only here can we say that the successful exercise of the authority of technical competence has occurred; as the scientist persuades his colleagues by his evidence and logic, so has the practitioner persuaded his client.

However, the alternative desired—even demanded—by the profession is that the client obey because he has faith in the competence of his consultant without evaluating the grounds of the consultant's advice. Indeed, members of consulting occupations attempt to avoid persuading their client to follow their advice. In medicine, such persuasion is invidiously labeled "selling oneself." Stress is placed on the necessity of faith or trust in the practitioner—in short, on *imputed* rather than demonstrated competence. A professional's advice should be obeyed because it is a professional who gives it, not because the advice is or can be evaluated on its evidential merits. Here we find the special source of the authority of the profession—incumbency in an expert status.

The Significance of "Free Choice"

The doctrine of "free choice," so prominent in the official ideology of medicine and other well-established professions, constitutes a device that allows the consultant to insist on faith and to practice on a take-it-or-leave-it basis markedly different from the way the scientist is obliged to "practice." The doctrine is, of course, designed to prevent "unfair competition" among practitioners by leaving the client free to choose among all of them. It is more generally justified by its protection of the client's own freedom. It may also be considered to be connected with the idea that consulting an expert is supposed to be a voluntary act on the part of the client. But it is perhaps less frequently recognized that the doctrine of free choice of services protects the consultant fully as much as it does the client. The expert may say, "After all, Mr. Jones, nobody is making you come to me, and I can't force you to take my advice. If you don't want to cooperate, go somewhere else."

In essence, the doctrine allows the consultant to put the burden of compliance on the client and to avoid the burden of having himself to persuade the client that compliance is in his interest. Indeed, it allows the consultant to disclaim any responsibility for persuading the client to take his advice. It allows him, in short, to rest on the authority of his professional status without having to try to present persuasive evidence to the client that his findings and advice are correct. It seems no accident that in any profession one working definition of success is the attainment of such prestige that one need not deal with anyone who does not come in as an humble supplicant eager to obey; it is the young practitioner and the comparative failure who must cope with the questioning.[13]

Two Levels of Professional Authority

Thus, in science the practitioner must attempt to influence others by the persuasiveness of the evidence supporting his assertions. But the institutional arrangements of that special group of consulting experts called professionals all function to minimize the necessity to influence by persuasion. In the case of the scientist, evidence of the technical competence used in reaching any concrete recommendation is required. In the case of the physician, the only evidence required is of being a bona fide expert. In this sense, the role of technical competence in professional authority is considerably different from technical competence in scientific authority.

It may seem peculiar and perverse to arrive at such a conclusion, for what is important about a profession if not some kind of technical competence, and why should one voluntarily put one's life, one's property, or one's soul in the hands of a man if he presents no evidence that he is competent to save it? It is precisely the running together of these two questions that confuses our understanding of the issues, for the question about competence asks why the governing bodies of societies decide to institutionalize the position of an occupation, while the other asks why individual clients obey individual members of an occupation.

In the former case we analyze public interaction at the centers of power between society's political establishment and the leaders of an occupation; in the latter we analyze the private interaction in local community settings between a variety of clients and practitioners. The qualities of the participants differ markedly in each case and so does the content of their interaction.

Surely the constitution of a profession by society should not be confounded with the work of individual practitioners. It seems quite correct to characterize as persuasion the way the leaders of an occupation influence the establishment to create and maintain it as a profession. This is how what Hughes called the "license and mandate" of the profession are obtained.[14] The leaders of an occupation persuade leaders of society that its members possess some technical competence so special and of such importance that the public should be prevented from using any other occupation with the same domain but assertedly less competence or integrity. The formal, institutionalized status of profession is granted by society on the basis of having been persuaded that an occupation is competent and responsible.

The interaction between client and practitioner is another matter. In practice, as I have tried to show, the typical form of influence is not to persuade the client of the competence of advice on the basis of available evidence, but rather to close off alternatives to him so that he has little choice but to go to the practitioner and to rely upon the authority of incumbency in a status to which competence has been imputed. It is the status that the compliant client relies on as evidence of competence, and it is the authority of incumbency that the practitioner prefers to assert. On a broad, societal level, then, a profession must persuade the sovereign of its competence. On the level of practice, competence is merely an imputation to the status of the individual professional, a status similar to that of the bureaucratic official.

Professional and Scientific Authority

I have argued that in the course of everyday work quite different kinds of "authority" are exercised by the scientist and by the professional owing to the quite different kinds of problems posed by the work of each. That the two presumably have in common some special esoteric knowledge or craft is far less important to their "authority" than that one works with colleagues and the other with laymen. It is this difference in the typical interactional contingencies of work that led Hughes to use the word "profession" in a way that excluded scientists and many other high-prestige occupations requiring intensive education and said to possess some special knowledge but which neither typically interact with lay clients nor possess extensive formal institutional sanctions.

Of course the usage of no word is sacred; the criterion of one's choice of usage must be its analytical value. Some sociologists have used the word "profession" to represent a college-educated segment of the labor force—what might be called buttoned-down-collar workers.[15] Naturally, such a usage has no value for discriminating *among* different occupations whose members are college-educated, from librarians to lawyers, executives to engineers. Many other sociologists have used the word "profession" in a more narrow sense but still broadly enough to include both scientists and the established consulting professions.[16] But, as has been demonstrated here, to ignore the difference between work on an everyday basis with a lay clientele and work in which one contends solely with colleagues confounds variations that have major analytical implications for the kind of authority that can be exercised in the course of work. So long as one must work with a lay clientele, the very fact that it *is* a lay clientele means that authority is problematic. The profession is the most successful and aspired-to consulting expert status precisely because it has achieved a stable institutional solution to the problem. And it is because it has achieved such a solution that the nature of the authority it wields in the course of everyday work is so very different from that of science. The authority of the professional is thus, in everyday practice, more like that of an officeholder than conventional characteristics would have us believe.

Finally, it seems appropriate to note that individuals can be *both* professionals and scientists—the physician, for example, seeing patients and doing research, the physicist doing research and consulting. This empirical fact does not vitiate the value of the distinction any more than does the fact that married men can be husbands and fathers at the same time discourage the distinction between these roles. Like the distinction between husband and father, the distinction between scientist and professional is made definite and stable by its emphasis on social relationships. Despite the fact that special knowledge and competence may be common to both, as masculinity is common to husband and father, the different relationships have consequences that ramify into such critical aspects of everyday work as the kind of authority that can be exercised. The distinction leads us to recognize those consequences, to emphasize not such a disembodied abstraction as advanced "education" or "knowledge," but rather the structure of human relationships that determines the way knowledge can be used. As I have shown in the case of the practicing profession of medicine, the application of knowledge is characteristically sustained by a form of authority that sets limits on the freedom of choice of the client, and this authority is more like that of the bureaucrat than that of the scientific expert.

NOTES

1. Everett Cherrington Hughes, *Men and Their Work* (Glencoe, Ill.: The Free Press, 1958), pp. 54–55.
2. *Ibid.*, p. 141.
3. *Ibid.*, p. 54.
4. *Ibid.*, p. 142.
5. Talcott Parsons, "Introduction," in Max Weber, *The Theory of Social and Economic Organization* (New York: Oxford University Press, 1947), p. 59.
6. See the notion of paradigm in Thomas Kuhn, *The Structure of Scientific Revolutions* (Chicago: University of Chicago Press, 1962).
7. See Hughes's discussion of psychology in these terms, *Men and Their Work*, pp. 139–144. See also the discussion of William J. Goode, "Encroachment, Charlatanism, and the Emerging Profession: Psychology, Sociology, and Medicine," *American Sociological Review*, 25 (1960), 902–914.
8. Gerald D. Berreman, "Brahmins and Shamans in Pahari Religion," *The Journal of Asian Studies*, 23 (1964), 67.
9. "He must be clean in person, well dressed, and anointed with sweet-smelling unguents that are not in any way suspicious." *Hippocrates* tr. W. H. S. Jones, "Loeb Classical Library" (Cambridge: William Heinemann, 1943), Vol. 2, p. 311.
10. Douglas Guthrie, "King James the Fourth of Scotland: His Influence on Medicine and Science," *Bulletin of the History of Medicine*, 21 (1947), 180–183.
11. This is the kernel of truth in Assemblyman Haskel's speech of 1834 urging the repeal of the New York State medical regulatory act: "Intrinsic merit . . . is the only qualification which ought to be required for any man to entitle him to practice physic or surgery." (Alex Berman, "The Thompsonian Movement and Its Relation to American Pharmacy and Medicine," *Bulletin of the History of Medicine*, 25 [1951], 422). And in

the matter of religion, this is the rationale underlying the rejection of the sanctity of sacraments administered by a properly ordained but personally sinful man as argued by, for example, the Donatists of the first millennium A.D.

12. Historical and contemporary variations in client relations in medicine are presented in Eliot Freidson, *Patients' Views of Medical Practice* (New York: Russell Sage Foundation, 1961).
13. This also seems to be a significant attribute of specialization and institutional practice—what I have called colleague-dependent practice in the last chapter. In medicine the specialist as well as the institutional practitioner has less need to be persuasive to his lay clientele than to his colleagues. There is some evidence that this is one of the attractions of such practice.
14. Hughes, *Men and Their Work*, pp. 78–87.
15. See, for example, William A. Faunce and Donald A. Clelland, "Professionalization and Stratification Patterns in an Industrial Community," *American Journal of Sociology*, 72 (1967), 341–350.
16. See, for example, William A. Kornhauser, *Scientists in Industry* (Berkeley: University of California Press, 1962).

5

Professional Dominance and the Ordering of Health Services

In the last chapter I pointed out that some but not all problems of authority in the doctor–patient relationship are managed if not solved by reliance upon the legally or otherwise formally created position of the profession—a position granted a monopoly over a set of services and the accessories they require. That position stands independently of the individual practitioner; it is as real as an ecological niche, and, like an ecological niche, the number and kinds of activities possible within it are limited. As a variable influencing the outcome of the consultative relationship it is separate and distinct from those of medical education (which is designed to influence the way individual physicians behave toward their patients) and from those of health education (which is designed to influence the way individual laymen behave toward themselves and toward consultation with physicians). It is a structural variable limiting the possibilities for behavior of the individuals involved, a variable reflecting the position of the medical profession in a formal system of organized consultative services.

But the position of the profession has significance that extends considerably beyond the guidance and limitation of interaction in consultation between doctor and patient. The structural position of the medical profession also patterns the relationships among a variety of other occupations that provide health-related services. Just as an ecological niche cannot be defined in and of itself but must instead be defined by its relation to the other niches of the total system, so the position of the profession must be defined by its relation to the other health workers in the system. In this chapter the relation of the profession to other occupations in health-related areas will be explored in an attempt to show that the nature of the medical profession's occupational position is such as to order a great deal of the total environment of medical care both within and outside treatment. In doing so, I shall use the concept of division of labor in a way that is not conventional in sociology; I shall treat it as a social organization of interrelated occupational groups that divides among them in an orderly way a complex of work activities. Thus, I shall treat the division of labor as an organized social structure. In order to dramatize the structural characteristics of the health-related division of labor I shall compare them with those of formally constituted bureaucratic organization. I shall point out that whereas in much of modern life the organizing principle of bureaucracy is an important source of social order that is thought to lead to client and worker dissatisfaction, the division of labor around health services, organized by the principle of professional dominance, provides an order similar to that of bureaucracy and seems to be as responsible for the pathologies of the system as is bureaucracy.

Bureaucracy and Profession

For at least a century we have been treated to the use of the word "bureaucracy" as an epithet. Indeed, we have tended to take as self-evidently true the assertion that the rationalization and systematization of work, governed by formal administrative authority and written rules, lead to a fragmentation of experience and a loss of meaning, a sense of alienation.[1] Bureaucratic principles have come to dominate the process of industrial production and increasingly dominate the commercial organization of sales and many personal services. Even more recently, in the case of health, education, and social welfare services, bureaucratization has been growing. In such settings, too, where the organization justifies its existence by the benefits it provides clientele, clients are said to suffer a sense of helplessness, anxiety, and resentment over the way the organization of services has led to depersonalization of their lives and loss of dignified identity. The culprit is thought to be the organizing principle of bureaucracy—orderly, systematic administrative procedures designed to ensure that work is done efficiently, honestly, and fairly.

In contrast to the negative word "bureaucracy" we have the word "profession." This word is almost always positive in its connotation, and is frequently used to represent a superior alternative to bureaucracy. Unlike "bureaucracy," which is disclaimed by every organization concerned with its public relations, "profession" is claimed by virtually every occupation seeking to improve its public image. When the two terms are brought together, the discussion is almost always at the expense of bureaucracy and to the advantage of profession. The principles underlying the two are said to be antithetical, the consequences of one being malignant and the other benign.

Over the years the literature has emphasized the difference between the two. Parsons pointed out that in his classic discussion of rational-legal bureaucracy Max Weber failed to distinguish between the authority of administrative office (generic to rational-legal bureaucracy) and the authority of expertise (generic to profession).[2] Making use of that distinction in the context of a study of a gypsum plant, Gouldner suggested that conventional, monocratic, and "punishment-centered" bureaucratic rules may not be as effective in ordering human effort in organizations as rules based on expertise and consented to by all parties involved.[3] Elaborating on Gouldner's discussion, Goss[4] and Smigel[5] have developed concepts of "advisory" and "professional" bureaucracy in which expertise is critical in creating and enforcing the rules. Many other writers, Thompson[6] and Blau[7] among them, have suggested that the principles of expertise and professionalization may constitute more efficient and more personally satisfying modes of organizing work than the classical principles of rational–legal administrative coordination. Expertise and professions are equated by virtually all writers, with a flexible, creative, and equalitarian way of organizing work, while bureaucracy is associated with rigidity and mechanical and authoritarian ways. There are, however, two important problems overlooked by that literature.

First, it seems to be assumed that technical expertise, unlike "arbitrary" administrative authority, is in some way neutrally functional and therefore so self-evidently true as to automatically produce cooperation or obedience in others as well as the efficient attainment of ends. In Gouldner's analysis, for example, we are told that as long as the *end* of technical expertise is accepted by workers, the expert's recommendation of means to that end will also be accepted automatically, or at least without serious question, in a "representative" or "expert" bureaucracy.[8] The implication is that when all workers can participate in setting ends in a complex organization, technical expertise can guide the way production is carried out without the necessity of exercising "punishment-centered" authority. Similarly, the implication in Parsons' comparison[9] of the authority of office with the authority of expertise is that while the former arbitrarily compels obedience, the latter is in some way naturally compelling by virtue of the fact that expertise and not office gives "orders."

But as I have shown in the preceding chapter, the authority of expertise is in fact problematic, requiring in its pure functional form the time-consuming and not always successful effort of persuading others that its "orders" are appropriate. As a special kind of occupation, professions have attempted to solve the problem of persuasion by obtaining institutional powers and prerogatives that at the very least set limits on the freedom of their prospective clients and that on occasion even coerce their clients into compliance. The expertise of the professional is institutionalized into something similar to bureaucratic office. The implications of this fact have not been considered in the literature comparing "bureaucratic" and "professional" modes of organizing the performance of work.

Second, virtually all past work has compared all specialized tasks organized by bureaucratic administration to the way members of a single specialized work group or profession within that larger organization are ordered by their occupational norms. Such comparison illogically contrasts a part with a whole. What is logically required is comparison between (1) the ordering and mobilization of *all* types of workers in the organization's division of labor by officeholders who have administrative but not necessarily technical or productive expertise, and (2) the ordering of the *complete* division of labor in an organization by the principle of technical expertise independent of bureaucratic office.

As I shall point out in this chapter, when one characterizes rational–legal monocratic bureaucracies as wholes, looks at the *total* collection of workers among whom professionals are found in some organizations, and examines how their interrelations are ordered by the authority of professional expertise, one finds distinctive properties that qualify considerably the significance of traditional contrasts between the consequences of bureaucracy and of profession on the experience of both workers and clients and on the distribution of services to clients. I wish to suggest that the division of labor has a social organization distinct from any external or artificial authority imposed on it by administrators. That social organization is constituted by the relations that occupations within a division of labor have to one another. Such relations are not only determined by the functional interdependence of those occupations but also by the formal social relationships of the occupations themselves. The social organization of the division of labor is especially distinctive, I believe, when occupations with a special professional status are involved. Indeed, a division of labor ordered by professional rather than by administrative authority contains within it mechanisms and consequences similar to those described as the pathologies of bureaucracy.

Concentrating on the field of health, which is the most highly professionalized area of work to be found in our society, I shall suggest that many of the rigid, mechanical, and authoritarian attributes, and much of the inadequate coordination said to characterize the health services, may stem more from their professional organization than from their bureaucratic characteristics. I shall discuss the influence of such organization on client experience as well as on the division of labor as such. Starting with a concrete organizational setting, I shall point out how one kind of professional organization produces a nonbureaucratic but nonetheless real rigidity and authoritarianism which may be as much if not more responsible for the tribulations of the patient than the specifically bureaucratic elements of the health organization. Furthermore, I will point out how the place of the dominant profession in the health-related division of labor influences other workers, the emphasis of health services, and the facility with which the client receives services. But I must first clarify what I mean by the word "profession."

Profession as Organized Autonomy

A great many words have been spoken in discussions of what a profession is, or rather, what the best definition of "profession" is. Unfortunately, discussion has been so fixed on the question of definition that not much analysis has been made of the significance and consequences of some of the elements common to most definitions. The most critical of such underexamined elements are organizational in character and are related to the organization of practice and the division of labor. Such elements are critical because they deal with facets of professional occupations that are independent of individual motivation or intention, and that may, as Carlin has suggested for law,[10] minimize the importance to behavior of the personal qualities of intelligence, ethicality, and trained skill imputed to professionals by most definitions. The key to such institutional elements of professions, I believe, lies in the commonly invoked word "autonomy." Autonomy means "the quality or state of being independent, free, and self-directing."[11] In the case of professions, autonomy apparently refers most of all to control over the content and the terms of work. That is, the professional is self-directing in his work.

From the single condition of self-direction or autonomy I believe we can deduce or derive virtually all the other institutional elements that are included in most definitions of professions. For example, an occupational group is more likely to be self-directing in its work when it has obtained a legal or political position of privilege that protects it from encroachment by other occupations. This is one of the functions of licensure, which provides an occupation with a legal monopoly over the performance of some strategic aspect of its work and effectively prevents free competition from other occupations. In the United States, for example, the physician is virtually the only one who can legally prescribe drugs and cut into the body. Competitors are left with being able to talk to patients and to lay hands *on* the body, but they may not penetrate the body chemically or physically.

Second, an occupational group is not likely to be able to be self-directing if it cannot control the production and particularly the application of knowledge and skill in the work it performs. This is to say, *if* the substance of its knowledge and skill is known to and performed by others, the occupation cannot be completely autonomous because those others can legitimately criticize and otherwise evaluate the way it carries out its work. The extended period of education controlled by the profession in an exclusively segregated professional school rather than in a variegated liberal arts school and a curriculum that includes some *special* theoretical content (whether scientifically proven or not) may represent a declaration that there is a body of special knowledge and skill necessary for the occupation that is not presented in colleges of arts and sciences or their specialized departments. The existence of such self-sufficient schools in itself rules out as *legitimate* arbiters of the occupation's work those with specialized training in the same area who received their training from some other kind of school. The professional school and its curriculum, of course, also constitute convenient institutional criteria for licensure, registration, or other exclusionary legal devices.

Third, a code of ethics or some other publicly waved banner of good intentions may be seen as a formal method of declaring to all that the occupation can be trusted, and so of persuading society to grant the special status of autonomy. The very existence of such a code implies that individual members of the occupation have the personal qualities of professionalism, the imputation of which is also useful for obtaining autonomy. Thus, most of the commonly cited attributes of professions may be seen either as consequences of their autonomy or as conditions useful for persuading the public and the body politic to grant such autonomy.

Autonomy and Dominance in the Division of Labor

Clearly, however, autonomy is not a simple criterion. One can think of many occupations that are autonomous merely by virtue of the esoteric character of their craft or the circumstances in which they work. Nightclub magicians and circus acrobats, for example, form autonomous occupations by virtue of their intensive specialization in an area of work that is itself narrowly specialized without at the same time constituting part of an interdependent division of labor. Other occupations, like cab drivers or lighthouse keepers, are fairly autonomous because their work takes place in a mobile or physically segregated context that prevents others from observing, and therefore evaluating and controlling, performance. In all these cases we have *autonomy by default.* An occupation is left wholly to its own devices because there is no strong public concern with its work, because it works independently of any functional division of labor, and because its work (in complexity, specialization, or observability) precludes easy evaluation and control by others. Where we find autonomy by default, we find no formal institutions in existence that serve to protect the occupation from competition, intervention, evaluation, and direction by others. Should interest in such an autonomous occupation be aroused among other workers or in society, its autonomy would prove to be fragile indeed without the introduction of such institutions. In short, *organized autonomy* is most stable and relevant to professions.

When we look at occupations engaged in such a complex division of labor as is found in the field of health, however, we find that with the exception of dentistry the only occupation that is truly autonomous is medicine itself.[12] It has the authority to direct and evaluate the work of others without in turn being subject to formal direction and evaluation by them. Paradoxically, its autonomy is sustained by the *dominance* of its expertise in the division of labor. It is true that some of the occupations it dominates—nursing for example—claim to be professions, as do other groups that lack either organized autonomy or dominance, such as schoolteachers and social workers. But surely there is a critically significant difference between dominant professions and those others that claim the name but do not possess the status. While the members of all may be committed to their work, may be dedicated to service, and may be specially educated, the dominant profession stands in an entirely different structural relationship to the division of labor than does the subordinate profession. To ignore that difference is to ignore something major. One might call many occupations "professions" if one so chooses, but there is a difference between the dominant profession and the others. In essence, the difference reflects the existence of a *hierarchy of institutionalized expertise*. That hierarchy of expertise, which is almost as definite as the hierarchy of office to be found in rational–legal monocratic bureaucracies,[16] can have the same effect on the experience of the client as bureaucracy is said to have. Let me briefly indicate how.

The Client in the Health Organization

Unlike education, where most services are given within complex organizations, most personal services in the field of health have been given in settings that are, organizationally, analogous to small shops. For a number of reasons, however, the proportion of personal health services given in complex organizations like hospitals seems to be increasing. It is the service in these complex organizations that has been most criticized for dehumanizing care, but is it bureaucratic office or institutionalized expertise that produces the client experience underlying that criticism?

Some complaints, like the cost of hospitalization, reflect the method of financing medical care in the United States rather than organization as such. Other complaints—such as those about poor food, noise, and general amenities—reflect the economic foundation and capital plant of the institution rather than its organization. For our present question, two sets of complaints seem most important—those related to the physical treatment for sickness and those related to the discomforts of being in a patient role in medical organizations.

Clearly, many complaints about the depersonalization of the client in the medical organization concern what some technical, ostensibly therapeutic, procedures do to people.[14] Simply to be strapped on a rolling table and wheeled down corridors, into and out of elevators, and, finally, into an operating room for the scrutiny of all is to be treated like an object, not a person. To be anesthetized is to become literally an object without the consciousness of a person. And to be palpated, poked, dosed, purged, cut into, probed, and sewed is to find oneself an object. In such cases, it is the technical work of the profession, not bureaucracy, that is responsible for some of the unpleasantness the client experiences in health organizations. That unpleasantness is partly analogous to what the industrial worker suffers when the machine he works on requires him to make limited, repetitive motions at some mechanically paced speed. It is directly analogous to what is suffered by the raw materials shaped by worker and machine in industry.

Such discomfort may easily be excused by the outcome—that is, improvement or cure is generally thought to be a product well worth the discomfort of being treated like an object. The problem, though, is to determine exactly how much of that treatment has any necessary bearing at all on the technical outcome. There is no doubt that some of the management of the patient has little or no bearing on the purely technical requirements for treatment.[15] Some practices bear on the bureaucratic problem of administering services to a number of individuals in a manner that is fair, precise, predictable, and economical. Other practices bear on the convenience of the staff, medical or otherwise, and while they may be justified by reference to staff needs as workers, such justification has no bearing on staff expertise as such. Without denying the role of formal bureaucratic organization in creating some of the problem, it is the role of the professional worker himself I wish to examine more closely, if only because, in medical and other organizations, the professional worker is specifically antibureaucratic, insisting on controlling the management of treatment himself. The question is, how do professional practices contribute to the unhappy experience of the patient?

The best way of beginning to answer this question lies in recalling the distinction I made between an object and a person. An object does not possess the capacity for understanding, and its behavior cannot be influenced by its understanding. When a person is treated *as if* he were an object, he will nonetheless behave on the basis of his understanding of that treatment. Naturally, his understanding is formed in part by what he brings with him into the treatment setting. It is also formed by the sense he himself can make of what is happening to him in the treatment setting. Since the treatment setting is presumably dominated by specialized, expert procedures, however, the most critical source of his information and understanding lies in the staff and its ability and inclination to communicate with the patient. If the staff does not communicate to the patient the meaning of and justification for what is done to him, it in essence refuses him the status of a responsible adult or of a person in the full sense of the word.

The extent to which the staff withholds information from the patient and avoids communicative interaction with him has been a common criticism of the operation of such medical organizations as hospitals.[16] The complaint is that no one tells the client what is going to be done to him, why, and when. And after he has been treated no one tells him why he feels the way he does, what can be expected subsequently, and whether or not he will live or die. The charge is that so little information is provided him that the patient cannot evaluate why he is being treated in a certain manner. Experience is mysteriously meaningless when it includes long waits for something unknown to happen or for something that does not happen, being awakened for an apparently trivial reason, being examined by taciturn strangers who enter the room unintroduced, perceiving lapses in such routines as medication and feeding without knowing whether error or intent is at issue. Surely this experience is little different from that of Kafka's antibureaucratic hero of *The Castle*.

Explanation by the staff constitutes acknowledgment of the client's status as a responsible adult capable of intelligent choice and self-control. In commercial organizations such acknowledgment does oocur, however superficially, by "personalized" forms. Why does it not occur in hospitals? Part of the reason may stem from the necessity to treat clients in batches standardized by their technical status and by the services required. Some reason may also be found in understaffing and overwork, which excuses the minimization of interaction with some in order to maximize it with those with more "serious" problems. But these reasons do not explain why *bureaucratic* solutions to the problem of communication are not adopted—for example, distributing brochures explaining and justifying hospital routines, describing the experience of "typical" cholycystectomies, mastectomies, or heart patients from the first day through convalescence, and including answers to "commonly asked questions." The prime reason for the failure to communicate with the patient does not, I believe, lie in under-financing, understaffing, or bureaucratization. Rather, it lies in the professional organization of the hospital and in the professional's conception of his relation to his clients.

Professional Control of Information

In the medical organization the medical profession is dominant. This means that all the work done by other occupations and related to the service of the patient is subject to the order of the physician.[17] The profession alone is held competent to diagnose illness, treat or direct the treatment of illness, and evaluate the service. Without medical authorization little can be done for the patient by paraprofessional workers. The client's medication, diet, excretion, and recreation are all subject to medical orders. So is the information given to the patient. By and large, without medical authorization paramedical workers are not supposed to communicate anything of significance to the patient about what his illness is, how it will be treated, and what the chances are for improvement. The physician himself is inclined to be rather jealous of the prerogative and is not inclined to authorize other workers to communicate information to the patient. Consequently, the paraprofessional worker who is asked for information by a patient is inclined to pass the buck like any bureaucrat. "You'll have to ask your doctor," the patient is told.

The dominant professional, then, is jealous of his prerogative to diagnose and forecast illness, holding it tightly to himself. But while he does not want anyone else to give information to the patient, neither is he himself inclined to do so. A number of reasons are advanced for this disinclination—the difficulty of being sure about diagnosis and precise about prognosis being perhaps the most neutral and technical of them all. Another reason is the physician's own busy schedule; he does not have the time to talk with the patient, and more serious cases need his attention. But the reasons of uncertainty and time-pressure are rather too superficial to dwell on. In the former case, the fact of uncertainty can constitute communication, though as Davis has shown[18] it can be asserted to avoid communication; in the latter case, surely the task can be delegated if time is lacking the doctor. For our present purposes, the most revealing argument against communication is based on characteristically professional assumptions about the nature of their clients. The argument, which goes back at least as far as Hippias' defensive remarks in the Hippocratic Corpus, asserts that, lacking professional training, the client is too ignorant to be able to comprehend what information he gets and that he is, in any case, too upset at being ill to be able to use the information he does get in a manner that is rational and responsible.[19] From this it follows that giving information to the patient does not help him, but rather upsets him and creates additional "management problems" for the physician. Thus, the patient should not be treated like an adult, but rather like a child, given reassurance but not information. To do otherwise would only lead to the patient being upset and making unnecessary trouble for the staff. Characteristically, the professional does not view the client as an adult, responsible person.

In addition, it is worth pointing out the implications of the professional insistence on faith or trust rather than persuasion. The client, lacking professional training, is thought to be unequipped for intelligent evaluation or informed cooperation with his consultant. Essentially, he is expected either to have faith in his consultant and do what he is told without searching question or else to choose another consultant in whom he does have faith. To question one's doctor is to show lack of faith and is justifiable grounds for the doctor to threaten to withdraw his services. Such insistence on faith, I believe, rests on more than the purely functional demands of an effective therapeutic or service relationship. It also neutralizes threat to status. The very special social position of institutionalized privilege that is the profession's is threatened as well as demeaned by the demand that advice and action be explained and justified to a layman. If he must justify himself to a layman, the professional must use grounds of evidence and logic common to both professional and layman and cannot use esoteric grounds known and subscribed to by the profession alone. Insistence on faith constitutes insistence that the client give up his role as an independent adult and, by so neutralizing him, protect the esoteric foundation of the profession's institutionalized authority.[20]

Other Workers in the Professional Organization

Thus far I have pointed out that in medical organizations, the source of a client's alienation is professional rather than bureaucratic authority.[21] Some alienating characteristics of professional authority may lead to practices with a curiously bureaucratic look to them, including such notorious practices as passing the buck and such a notorious problem as (in the form of requiring doctors' orders) red tape. In this organization the client's position is similar to his position in civil service bureaucracies—he is handled like an object, given little information or opportunity for choice, and made to feel less than a responsible adult. And what of the subordinate worker in this setting dominated by a profession?

As noted in the beginning of this chapter, many writers have felt that the worker as well as the client suffers from the bureaucratization of production by a monocratic administration. Lacking identification with the prime goals of the organization, lacking an important voice in setting the formal level and direction of work, and performing work that has been so rationalized as to become mechanical and meaningless, a minute segment of an intricate mosaic of specialized activities that he is in no position to perceive or understand, the worker is alienated. In contrast to the bureaucratized worker, however, the professional is said to be committed to and identified with his work so that it retains meaning for him, becoming in fact a central life interest. This may be true for dominant professions, but what of the other occupations working in the organization that the professional dominates? Are they not prone to alienation?

By and large, this question has not been asked in past studies, for the emphasis has been more on the positive response of "professionalism" than on the negative responses of alienation. What evidence there is, however, indicates that there are serious problems of worker morale in professional settings. Available studies are fairly clear about the existence of hierarchy in the professional health organization and about a decrease of participation in decision making the farther down the hierarchy one goes. Neither the ends nor the means of their work seem to be a matter for legitimate determination by lower-level workers, though, of course, they do sometimes have a very strong informal influence on such determination. Furthermore, even in situations where the stated official expectation is free participation by all workers in conferences about the running of such units as wards, participation has been observed to be quite unequal.[22]

The paraprofessional worker is, then, like the industrial worker, subordinated to the authority of others. He is not, however, subordinated solely to the authority of bureaucratic office, but also to the putatively superior knowledge and judgment of professional experts. In some studies this authority is characterized as a kind of stratification,[23] in others as a function of status.[24] In very few, if any, studies is that status or stratification said to be of administrative or bureaucratic origin. It is instead largely of professional origin. In a few studies the notion of alienation has been specifically cited.[25] Clearly, while there is no comparative evidence to allow us to determine whether more or fewer workers are alienated from professional than from bureaucratic organizations, neither hierarchical nor authoritarian tendencies are missing in the professional organization of the division of labor, nor are alienation, absenteeism, low morale, and high turnover insignificant problems. It is as true for the worker as for the patient that the professionally organized division of labor has pathologies similar to those stemming from bureaucracy.

Substantive Bias in Client Services

Thus far I have compared the influence of professional authority with the influence of bureaucratic authority on the experience of both client and worker in the physically limited corporate body we usually call an organization. However, because interorganizational relations may themselves be seen as organization and since the production of particular goods and services is rarely limited to the confines of a single corporate body requiring a variety of functions from outside "the" organization, it seems useful to continue my comparison in the rather broader context of planning and coordinating service as such. I have already noted that the common assumption is that expert authority has a neutral, functional foundation rather than, like bureaucratic authority, the foundation of arbitrary office. If this is so, we should expect the influence of expert authority on the support and planning of services to be highly functional, lacking arbitrary bias from the special vantage of bureaucratic office. Our expectation is not met in health services. There, the dominant profession exercises great influence on the disposition of resources that makes services available for clients. The character of that influence does stem from professional views of the purely functional considerations of what service is needed to accomplish some desired end, but *those views have been distorted by the lenses of a special occupational perspective.*

To understand how resources get distributed to the varied health services sought or required by the client, we must keep in mind the fact that the *medical* division of labor is not functionally complete. It is composed solely of those occupations and services controlled by the dominant profession. Outside it are some performing work that is functionally and substantively related to the profession but not subject to the profession's authority. In matters of health in the United States, such occupations as dentistry, optometry, chiropracty, and clinical psychology exemplify by their independent existence the functional incompleteness of the medically ordered division of labor. Furthermore, there are occupational groups whose work is often at least partly related to health problems but which are not recognized medical occupations; schoolteachers, specialized training and guidance personnel, social workers, and even ministers may be cited here. These are not part of the medically ordered division of labor either. Thus, while the profession stands as the supreme authority in the medical division of labor, the medical division of labor does not encompass all health-related activities of the larger health-related division of labor. Nonetheless, the distribution of support and resources tends to move disproportionately through the medical division of labor.

I have argued for the distinction of a type of profession that has ultimate authority over its work in such a way that it is self-directing or autonomous and dominant in a division of labor. In the case of medicine, a strategic facet of its authority is its delineation of pathology, the definitions of health and illness that guide the application of knowledge to human ills. The physician is the ultimate expert on what is health and what illness and on how to attain the former and cure the latter. Indeed, his perspective leads him to see the world in terms of health and illness, and the world is presently inclined to turn to him for advice on all matters related to health and illness regardless of his competence. Given the highly visible miracles medicine has worked over the past century, the public has even been inclined to ask the profession to deal with problems that are not of the biophysical character for which success was gained from past efforts. What were once recognized as economic, religious, and personal problems have been redefined as illness and have therefore become medical problems.[26] This widening of medical jurisdiction has had important consequences for the allocation of resources to client services.

No philanthropies today seem to be able to attract more financial support than those devoting themselves to illness, particularly those of children. If the label of illness can be attached to a problem it receives extensive support and also becomes dominated by medical institutions even when there is no evidence that medical institutions have any especially efficacious way of dealing with the problem. By virtue of controlling the notions of illness and health, medicine has in fact become a giant umbrella under which a disparate variety of workers (including sociologists) can be both financed and protected from overly close outside scrutiny merely through their semantic connection with health. But those who do not or cannot choose to huddle under the umbrella, even though their work is health-related, tend to find it difficult to obtain support.

One rather obvious consequence is the uneven distribution of resources to health-related activities. For example, it was pointed out recently that heavy financing has been given to medical research into mental deficiency, only a small amount of which is biologically or genetically caused, while *educational* facilities for the training and teaching of mental deficients have been sorely underfinanced.[27] Less obvious and more important to public welfare is the extent to which this uneven distribution of resources emphasizes some hypotheses and investigatory and therapeutic models at the expense of others equally plausible. For example, it was recently noted that work in rehabilitation has come under medical supervision, resulting in an inappropriate emphasis on the traditional authoritarian therapeutic relationship of medicine that I have already discussed.[28] It has also been noted that the disease model has dominated the approach to mental illness.[29] By and large, within the well-financed division of labor dominated by the profession and under its protective umbrella, most work is limited to that which conforms to the special perspective and substantive style of the profession—a perspective that emphasizes the individual over the social environment, the treatment of rare and interesting over common and uninteresting disorders, the cure rather than the prevention of illness, and preventive medicine rather than what might be called "preventive welfare"—social services and resources that improve the diet, housing, way of life, and motivation of the people without their having to undertake clinical consultation with a practitioner. In short, I suggest that by virtue of its position in the public esteem and in its own division of labor, the dominant profession of the field of health exerts a special and biased influence on planning and financing services of the general field within which it is located. The prime criterion for determining that emphasis is not necessarily functional in character, but social and structural—whether or not the services can be dominated by or be put under the umbrella of the dominant profession. The consequence for the client is an array of differentially supported services that may not be adequate for his needs and interests.

Finally, I might point out that given this array of health-related services differentially developed and supported by functional and other considerations, still further qualification of the kind of service a client is likely to get is exercised by the dominant profession. In general, I wish to suggest that when some of the relevant services lie outside the medical division of labor and some inside, serious problems of access to care and of the rational coordination of care are created by the barriers that the profession erects between that segment of the division of labor it does dominate and that segment it does not.[30]

Perhaps the simplest way of discussing these barriers is to examine the process by which clients move through the division of labor. They move in part by their own choice and selection of consultants and in part by their consultants' choice of and referral to other consultants or technicians. To the extent that the client moves through the division of labor by his own volition, he is responsible for his own care and his consultants are dependent on him for relevant information about his problem. But to the extent to which the client is being guided by consultants, the character of his experience and care is dependent on the substantive direction of his consultants' referrals and on the exchange of information bearing on treatment among them. Here is where the professionally created barrier is found. Within the general health division of labor, the referral of clients tends to go in only one direction—into the smaller medical division of labor, without also going from the medical into the larger system. This is also generally true of the transmission of information about the client. To put it more bluntly, teachers, social workers, ministers, and others outside the medical division of labor refer to physicians and communicate information about the client to them, but physicians are not likely either to refer clients to them or to provide them with the results of medical investigation.[31]

By the same token, physicians do not routinely refer to clinical psychologists, optometrists, chiropractors, and others outside the medical division of labor but clearly within the health division of labor. They are likely to refer only when they are sure that the limited services they may order—psychological testing rather than psychotherapy, spectacle fitting and sales rather than refractions, and minor manipulations for medically untreatable muscular–skeletal complaints rather than for other complaints—will be performed, and no more. They are also, wittingly or not, likely to discourage such workers' referrals to them by reciprocating neither referrals nor information about their findings. And from at least one study there is evidence that medically oriented workers are prone to reject the patient if he comes to them from the wrong source.[32]

By and large, physicians refer to and communicate extensively with only those who, within the medical division of labor, are subject to their prescription, order, or direction. Indeed, physicians are likely to be very poorly informed about any institutional and occupational resources that lie outside their own jurisdiction. And, as is quite natural for people who have developed commitment to their work, they are likely to be suspicious of the value of all that lies outside their domain, including the competence and ethicality of those working outside. Their commitment leads them to deprecate the importance of extramedical services, and their position as professionals encourages them to restrict their activities to the medical system they control. So long as this is all their clients need or want, no harm is done save for the possibility that the professional's response to outside services may encourage those outside to avoid or delay in referring clients to the physician. Even when outside services are necessary for the client's well-being, referral to them may be delayed or never undertaken and the client's interests left unprotected.

The Role of Professionalism

Its position in the health division of labor permits the medical profession to reinforce and protect itself from outside influence and to claim and maintain jurisdiction and control over many more areas than logic or evidence justifies. Why it uses its position the way it does, however, remains unexamined. Some critics seem prone to imply that professions are, in spite of their protestations, simply unconcerned with the public good and dominated by self-interest. However, it seems to me instead that professions have those weaknesses not because they are inherently venal but rather because like all institutions they are composed of men who must, in order to serve the institution, become deeply committed to the concrete works and days of *being* professionals. They must internalize the ideals of the institution and at the same time find a life in being a professional person and doing professional work. Their commitment to professional ideals and career is expressed in attitudes, ideas, and beliefs that might be called "professionalism." It is professionalism itself that seems to transform the ideal responsibility to serve the good of the general public into limited concrete responsibility to serve the good of one's personal public, and the ideal of universalistic knowledge and skill into particularistic sectarianism expressed by occupational imperialism. While the ideals are truly part of professionalism, they are only one part. Their interaction with other values connected with professionalism seems to produce such a transformation.

Professionalism seems to be composed of three major sets of attitudes, values, or orientations: one set addressed to the professional ideals of knowledge and service, one to the professional occupation and the life-career it provides, and one to the character of professional work. The first set is composed of the values conventionally ascribed to professionals—the ideals of professional institutions which are expressed by individual professionals as commitment to applying knowledge and skill unselfishly to the benefit of mankind. Such ideals have been found by empirical studies to exist among aspirants to the professions and are expressed concretely in survey questionnaires as interest in helping people, in the intellectual stimulation of work, and in being creative and original.[33]

Those idealistic professional values cannot stand alone in professionalism, however. They are abstract values by themselves, able to become real only when connected with the second set of values of professionalism—commitment to the occupation that itself defines and organizes the work. Students do not merely want to heal, to serve justice, or to transmit knowledge to the young; they want to be doctors, lawyers, or teachers. Their interest in becoming a member of a profession is the vehicle for their interest in serving mankind. And being committed to a particular occupation, of course, includes commitment to the costs and rewards of a particular occupational career. Work in the occupation, not work alone, becomes a central life interest.

The occupation being the source and focus of his commitment, the individual is naturally concerned with the prestige of the occupation and its position in the class structure and in the market place. Thus, empirical studies of undergraduate aspirants to the major professions find them to be not only interested in helping people and the like but also interested in the high income and prestige they expect from their professional careers.[34] Such findings seem to belie dedication and are treated by many analysts of professions with either silence or embarrassment. However, they express values that are as essential to professionalism as "ideals," for they commit men to the organized work activity by which ideals are realized.

Clearly, the very fact of occupational organization limits the perspective from which the professional's ideals can be seen and realized. Professionalism in medicine, for example, does not mean commitment to healing in the abstract, general sense of the word. There is only commitment to healing in the limited way the medical profession defines it. And commitment to serving mankind (or service orientation, as it is sometimes put) is limited to service in those ways the profession defines as being in the public interest. Operative professionalism is thus constituted by commitment to occupationally defined knowledge and technique and occupationally defined public service, to a particular occupation's view of correct knowledge and ethicality.

Finally, the third set of values of professionalism defines the character of the work to which one's career is devoted. Essentially, it defines the work to be extraordinarily complex and nonroutine, requiring for its adequate performance extensive training, great intelligence and skill, and highly complex judgment that cannot be evaluated by any straightforward and definite rules. The truth of that definition of work is, though not really established empirically, generally accepted by professional writers on the professions. Its truth is, however, irrelevant to understanding the important role it plays in professionalism and in the struggle to gain or maintain professional authority, autonomy, and prestige. *Belief* in the extraordinary character of the work and of the performer sustains the worker's claim that he must be able to exercise his own complex, individual judgment independently of others, that is, he must be independent and autonomous. While members of *most* occupations seek to be free to control the level and direction of their work efforts, it is distinct to professionalism to assert that such freedom is a necessary condition for the proper performance of work. And it is precisely such an emphasis on individual judgment and independence, founded on a conception of the character of the work, which allows the self-regulatory processes of professions to shift from the ideal of responsibility for the actions of one's colleagues to concrete responsibility for oneself, to shift from belief in the ideal of responsibility for the public good to the practice of responsibility for the good of one's own personal clientele.

Similarly, we can understand something of the roots of professional imperialism and narrowness by considering both this view of the character of work and its interaction with career commitment. The work being thought to be what it is, it follows that the man who is qualified to perform it must be himself a rather extraordinary, gifted person. And so are his colleagues and his profession. In conjunction with the ideals asserting the mission of his profession, this *professional pride* leads the worker to consider himself to be quite different from, indeed superior to, those of other occupations. Reinforced by the obvious material interest that commitment to occupational life-career inevitably involves, such a view of self seems likely to lead to downright suspicion of the competence and ethicality of all whose work is related to his but not subject to his evaluation and control. And when outsiders doing work related to his espouse a mission predicated upon a different set of paradigms than that of his profession, the professional rather naturally feels that they and their occupation should either be converted and controlled (as medicine seems to be doing to osteopathy), or, if not destroyed, excluded from any significant interaction. And so it is that the thrust of professional activity is to seek to build barriers that keep the profession and its clientele safe from those beyond the pale while at the same time seeking jurisdiction over all that cannot be excluded.

In essence, my argument has been that the weaknesses to be found in professions are not mere flaws that can be corrected by recruiting better men, improving their training, and organizing their work more effectively. They cannot be eradicated by the profession itself. Those weaknesses are consequences of the fact that men cannot be led to serve an occupation by becoming committed to its ideals alone. They must also become committed to a concrete career and to concrete, historically located institutions. And in the case of professionals they also develop a sense of pride based on a typical conception of the special nature of their work. All three things, I suggest, compose professionalism, and in their interaction they produce the characteristic weaknesses of professions. *And since those weaknesses stem from professionalism itself, professions cannot be expected to be able to rectify them.*

Profession, Bureaucracy, and the Client

I began this chapter with the comment that "bureaucracy" has become an epithet. From what I have said about "profession" in my exposition, one might think that I am attempting to make it an epithet also. This is not true. It is true, however, that I have attempted to remove the word from the realm of the normative, where most usage has been prone to keep it, and to move it into a realm subject to logical and empirical investigation. In this effort, I have chosen first to use the word to refer to a way of *organizing work* rather than, as is common, to refer to an *orientation* toward work or a body of *knowledge*. By that criterion I suggested that we might distinguish between what are commonly (and, I believe, meaninglessly) called professions and those professions that are dominant, directing others in a division of labor and being themselves autonomous, subject to direction by no other. Medicine is one of those dominant professions.

After discussing the implications of this usage for the other variables commonly attached to the notion of profession, I then went on to suggest some ways the medical profession influences health services. First, I suggested that the experience of the client in the medical organization—particularly the hospital—is created less by the bureaucratic elements in those organizations than by the work as such and by the perspective of the dominant profession that orders the activity of most of the occupations in the organization. Second, I suggested that the experience of the worker in the medical organization suggests alienation similar to that said to exist in bureaucratically organized settings. Third, I suggested that the planning and distribution of health resources tend to be weighted by the dominant profession's structural position in the division of labor as well as by the functional problems of health and illness as such. Finally, I suggested that in the cooperative exchange and referral of clients, which is a prerequisite for the expeditious delivery of all necessary health-related services, the physician neither reciprocates referrals nor communicates with those who work outside his own division of labor. In all four cases, and perhaps in more, I suggest, the relations between clients and the services they need are influenced strongly by the dominance of a single, autonomous profession. Insofar as there is pathology, much stems from the profession, not bureaucracy.

Thus, I suggest that the dominance of client services by the principle of expertise embodied in a professionally ordered division of labor is, analytically and practically, fully as problematic as dominance by the principles of rational–legal bureaucracy. Expertise institutionalized into a profession is not, as much writing seems to assume, an automatically self-correcting, purely task-oriented substitute for "arbitrary" bureaucracy. Expertise establishes office and hierarchy analogous to that of bureaucracy. The definition of the work—that is, how the client should behave and what other workers should do—is a partial expression of the hierarchy created by the office and of the ideology stemming from the perspective of the office as well as of the purely technical character of the work itself. And when that work involves personal services of some importance to the welfare of the client, both the ideology and the technology combine to produce bureaucracy-like consequences.

Limitations on the Professional Perspective

Finally, I may say that my intent here has not been to find villains on whom to blame the problems confronting the organization and presentation of client services. Consonant with my emphasis in this book, I refer to social structure rather than individual attributes. Both professional and bureaucrat have, by and large, the best of intentions. Both, like everyone else, are creatures of their perspectives, and those perspectives are limited by training, by commitment, and by personal work experience that comes to be regarded as wisdom. I attempted to show how, from the fact of being a professional worker, the perspective of professionalism arises to justify and impel much of professional performance. Such performance is not some easily remedied defect, but rather something inherent in the nature of social life that requires countervailing pressure from other perspectives more than better intentions from within. One serious difference between professional and bureaucrat, however, lies in the very existence of legitimate countervailing pressures.

As Parsons pointed out in distinguishing between the authority of office and the authority of expertise, a critical difference between bureaucrat and professional lies in the foundation for their authority. One is largely a creature of the organization itself and the laws that establish it, answerable to the organizational rules and to a legal order that stands outside him, his colleagues, and the organization in which he works. His client has recourse to both sets of rules and, in our society at least, has specific civil rights in that order. While a serious problem of our time is how we can make such a formal rational–legal order actually work efficiently, fairly, and humanely, the principles of the order are designed to protect both worker and client, giving them the basic right to be recognized as responsible adults.

Such protection does not exist unequivocally in professional organizations. Unlike the bureaucrat, who may on occasion attain autonomy *by default*, the professional has gained *organized autonomy* and is not bound by rules that stand outside his profession. His performance, however, can produce the same barriers to communication and cooperation within a functional division of labor, the same structures of evasion, and the same reduction of the client to an object which have been attributed to bureaucratic organization. In the name of health the client may be stripped of his civil status, a status which is as much if not more an element of his welfare than his health. But unlike bureaucratic practices, which in rational–legal orders are considered arbitrary and subject to appeal and modification, professional practices are imputed to have the unquestioned objectivity of expertise and scientific truth, and so are not routinely subject to higher review or change by virtue of outside appeal. There is no generally accepted notion of due process for the layman—client or worker—in professional organization. And in theory, the lack of review or due process is as it should be, since the professional's is not supposed to be the arbitrary authority of bureaucratic office. In practice in the everyday world, though, there is no such thing as pure knowledge or expertise—there is only knowledge in the service of a practice.

Here is the crux of the matter. Expertise is not mere knowledge. It is the practice of knowledge, organized socially and serving as the focus for the practitioner's commitment. In this sense, it is not merely mechanical skill which, like the cog of a machine, automatically fits itself into Durkheim's organic order. The worker does not see his work as merely different from another's. He develops around it an ideology and, with the best of intentions, an imperialism that stresses the technical superiority of his work and his capacity to perform it. This imperialistic ideology is built into the perspective that his training and practice create. It cannot be overcome by ethical dedication to the public interest because it is sincerely believed in as the only proper way to serve the public interest. And it hardens when an occupation develops the autonomy of a profession and a place of dominance in a division of labor and when expertise becomes an institutional status rather than a capacity. The pathology arises when outsiders may no longer evaluate the work by the rules of logic and the knowledge available to all educated men and when the only legitimate spokesman on an issue relevant to all men must be someone who is officially certified. This is the central policy issue in the provision of such personal services as health care, an issue underlying such concrete questions as how the services are to be paid for and how they are to be presented to the public. The issue is who is to determine what the goals of the service are and the concrete modes by which its goals are to be pursued.

In essence, my position is that the delivery of medical care cannot be controlled by the profession, that its autonomy and its dominance must be tempered by administrative or bureaucratic mechanisms that stress accountability for effective and humane services and must be in some way more responsive to the lay client himself. In Part III of this book I shall examine first hospitals and then ambulatory care services to show the consequences of professional rather than bureaucratic dominance. After that examination I shall be in a position to suggest ways by which medical services can be reorganized so as to create a more flexible and responsive environment for their delivery.

NOTES

1. For an excellent brief introduction see Peter Blau, *Bureaucracy in Modern Society* (New York: Random House, 1956).
2. Talcott Parsons, Introduction to Max Weber, *The Theory of Social and Economic Organization* (New York: Free Press, 1964), pp. 58–60.
3. Alvin W. Gouldner, *Patterns of Industrial Bureaucracy* (New York: Free Press, 1964).
4. Mary E. W. Goss, "Patterns of Bureaucracy among Hospital Staff Physicians," in Eliot Freidson, ed., *The Hospital in Modern Society* (New York: Free Press, 1963), pp. 170–194.
5. Erwin O. Smigel, *The Wall Street Lawyer* (New York: Oxford University Press, 1947).
6. Victor Thompson, *Modern Organization* (New York: Knopf, 1961).
7. Peter Blau, *The Dynamics of Bureaucracy* (Chicago: University of Chicago Press, 1959).
8. Gouldner, *Patterns of Industrial Bureaucracy*, pp. 221–222.
9. Parsons, Introduction to Weber's *Theory of Social and Economic Organization.*
10. Jerome Carlin, *Lawyers' Ethics* (New York: Russell Sage Foundation, 1966). It should be noted that Carlin's findings also were that a stable individual attribute of ethicality influenced behavior independently of the setting. A recent study of college students found the same thing. See William J. Bowers, "Normative Constraints on Deviant Behavior in the College Context," *Sociometry*, 31 (December, 1968), 370–385.
11. *Webster's Third New International Dictionary* (Springfield, Mass.: C. & C. Merriam Co., 1967), p. 148.
12. See Eliot Freidson, "Paramedical Personnel," in *International Encyclopedia of the Social Sciences* (New York: Macmillan and Free Press, 1968), Vol. 10, pp. 114–120, for more discussion on the medical division of labor.

13. A recent article argues persuasively against the value of using the idea of formal bureaucratic organization to analyze settings in which professionals work, pointing out that even in industrial settings the idea does not faithfully reflect observed behavior. See Rue Bucher and Joan Stelling, "Characteristics of Professional Organization," *Journal of Health and Social Behavior*, 10 (1969), 3–15. The same point may be made for the division of labor I describe. However, formal bureaucratic organization and formal occupational jurisdiction and authority do provide limits of a fairly definite nature; just as a stenographer cannot negotiate with her employer over who will chair a policy making meeting, so a nurse cannot negotiate with a surgeon over who will perform an operation.
14. Important in this context is Erving Goffman's "The Medical Model and Mental Hospitalization," in Erving Goffman, *Asylums* (Garden City, N. Y.: Doubleday, 1961), pp. 321–386.
15. For an extended analysis of the substance of expertise which tries to indicate what is genuine and what spurious in medical work, see Eliot Freidson, *Profession of Medicine: A Study of the Sociology of Applied Knowledge* (New York: Dodd-Mead, 1970), Chapter 15.
16. For example, see the following: Julius A. Roth, "The Treatment of Tuberculosis as a Bargaining Process," in A. M. Rose, ed., *Human Behavior and Social Processes* (Boston: Houghton Mifflin, 1962), pp. 575–588; Jeanne C. Quint, "Institutionalized Practices of Information Control," *Psychiatry*, 28 (1965), 119–132.
17. For example, see Albert F. Wessen, "Hospital Ideology and Communication Between Ward Personnel," in E. G. Jaco, ed., *Patients, Physicians, and Illness* (New York: Free Press, 1958), pp. 448–468.
18. Fred Davis, "Uncertainty in Medical Prognosis, Clinical and Functional," *American Journal of Sociology*, 66 (1960), 41–47.
19. See, for example, the material in Barney G. Glaser and Anselm L. Strauss, *Awareness of Dying* (Chicago: Aldine, 1965).
20. For a more extensive discussion of the professional ideology see Freidson, *Profession of Medicine*, Chapter 8.
21. For a rare study of patients using a measure of alienation, see John W. Evans, "Stratification, Alienation, and the Hospital Setting," *Engineering Experiment Station Bulletin* No. 184, Ohio State University, 1960.

22. For example, see the findings in William Caudill, *The Psychiatric Hospital as a Small Society* (Cambridge, Mass.: Harvard University Press, 1958), and William A. Rushing, *The Psychiatric Professions* (Chapel Hill: University of North Carolina Press, 1964), pp. 258–259.
23. See M. Seeman and J. W. Evans, "Stratification and Hospital Care," *American Sociological Review*, 26 (1961), 67–80, 193–204, and Ivar Oxaal, "Social Stratification and Personnel Turnover in the Hospital," *Engineering Experiment Station Monograph* No. 3, Ohio State University, 1960.
24. See E. G. Mishler and A. Tropp, "Status and Interaction in a Psychiatric Hospital," *Human Relations*, 9 (1956), 187–205, and William R. Rosengren, "Status Stress and Role Contradictions: Emergent Professionalization in Psychiatric Hospitals," *Mental Hygiene*, 45 (1961), 28–39.
25. See Rose L. Coser, "Alienation and the Social Structure: Case Study of a Hospital," in Freidson, *Hospital in Modern Society*, pp. 231–265, and L. I. Pearlin, "Alienation from Work: A Study of Nursing Personnel," *American Sociological Review*, 27 (1962), 314–326.
26. For an extended discussion of the relative place of notions of health and illness in modern society, see Freidson, *Profession of Medicine*, Chapter 12.
27. George W. Albee, "Needed—A Revolution in Caring for the Retarded," *Trans-action*, 5 (1968), 37–42.
28. Albert F. Wessen, "The Apparatus of Rehabilitation: An Organizational Analysis," in Marvin B. Sussman, ed., *Sociology and Rehabilitation* (Washington, D. C.: American Sociological Association, 1966), pp. 148–178.
29. See Marline Taber et al., "Disease Ideology and Mental Health Research," *Social Problems*, 16 (1969), 349–357, for a recent statement.
30. See the discussion in William L. Kissick, "Health Manpower in Transition," *The Milbank Memorial Fund Quarterly*, 46 (January 1968), Part 2, pp. 53–91, for this and many other relevant points.
31. For work bearing on these statements see Elaine Cumming et al., *Systems of Social Regulation* (New York: Atherton, 1968), and Eugene B. Piedmont, "Referrals and Reciprocity: Psychiatrists, General Practitioners, and Clergymen," *Journal of Health and Social Behavior*, 9 (1968), 29–41.

32. See David Schroder and Danuta Ehrlich, "Rejection by Mental Health Professionals: A Possible Consequence for Not Seeking Appropriate Help for Emotional Disorders," *Journal of Health and Social Behavior*, 9 (1968), 222–232.

33. Cf. Morris Rosenberg, *Occupations and Values* (New York: Free Press, 1957), and James A. Davis, *Great Aspirations* (Chicago: Aldine, 1964).

34. *Ibid.*

Part 3

PROBLEMS OF ORGANIZING MEDICAL CARE

6

Organizing Hospital Care

My premise is that in health services professional dominance is a sufficient problem to warrant the strengthening of management and of bureaucratic procedures. I am sure, however, that this elicits in the reader's mind the refrain, "Do not clip, mark, fold, tear, or staple this card." The IBM card, a polemical symbol of our time, represents the transformation of human beings for purposes of better administration. The services administered are usually supposed to benefit people, but in the course of being benefited they are transformed into ciphers, which, it is felt, is no benefit. Nonetheless, rationalization proceeds in all service industries. Such rationalization requires breaking services into standardized units. Traditional industrial sociology has concerned itself with what the rationalization of manufacturing has done to the worker (and vice versa). The new industrial sociology concerns itself with what the rationalization of services has done to the people getting them and why.

In Part II I discussed the professional foundation of such rationalization in health institutions and the relationship of bureaucratic or administrative rationalization to the process. In this and succeeding chapters I shall discuss the concrete organizations in which such rationalization has been taking place. Here I shall examine the hospital, which is one of the major institutions devoted to the processing of people thought to require health services. I shall not, however, concern myself with the technicalities of financing or administering hospitals.[1] Furthermore, I shall not address myself to the medical, and particularly the psychiatric, literature on what is thought to be therapeutic in hospital management. Consonant with the approach of this book, I shall emphasize the way various organizational arrangements influence the quality of staff and client experience in the service industry at issue here. I shall do so by reviewing the major sociological studies of hospitals that have been reported over the past fifteen years. And I shall argue that professional dominance creates sufficient problems to require the development of a stronger countervailing administrative management and of a better organized clientele.

In dealing with such health factories as hospitals, I deal with service industries. But may we speak of service industries generically, or must we distinguish them into significant types of service industries? Is the hospital fully comparable to a hotel, or the college campus to an amusement park? Partially so, but I think there are some critical differences. First, services competing with others in a relatively free consumer market must be distinguished from a service monopoly. Second, frankly profit-making services may be distinguished from nonprofit, ostensibly altruistic services. Taken together, the two simple distinctions may be used to discriminate between commercial and professionalized services. The distinctions are important for the customer because they point to different degrees of control over the selection of services that can be exercised by the recipient: whether he can choose *not* to use a service and whether he can freely choose among alternatives of service.

The hospital belongs to that growing segment of organized service industries in which a number of systematic barriers to free choice exists, and in which, instead of being a customer, the consumer becomes a pupil, a client, a patient, or otherwise a member of a flock. Here, the responsibility to be aware of his need for a service sometimes may be left to the customer, as well as some choice to use what is available, but as I have already noted, the market is not left free to provide all he may personally want. In health above all, but also in law, education, welfare, and to a degree religion, the market is restricted to that which is licensed, certified, accredited, or otherwise officially approved, and control over the definition of services is held by those who control the *production* of services rather than those who consume them.

Clearly, it is in this type of service industry that the fate of the consumer is most problematic. And it is rationalization in this type of service industry that has stimulated the most dismay and rebellion on the part of the contemporary American consumer and the most concern with reform on the part of society. Studies of hospitals reported by social scientists over the past fifteen years have faithfully reflected the problems of rationalizing noncommercial services and have brought out the nature of the problem of analysis and decision confronting us now. Let us look at some of those studies.

The Prevalence of Depersonalization

One theme of some importance in many studies is the depersonalization of the patient. In the residential establishments called total institutions, Goffman asserts that the individual's self is stripped, trimmed, mortified, defaced, and otherwise disfigured in the course of obtaining service.[2] Surely there is evidence of this in reports from mental hospitals in the United States,[3] homes for the aged in Great Britain,[4] and general hospitals.[5] But the problem is not of the same magnitude in all kinds of establishments. For example, tax-supported hospitals seem to regiment and depersonalize the patient more than private hospitals, and mental hospitals seem to strip and mortify patients considerably more than general hospitals.

The analytical factor common to both these contrasts is the status of the client. *Depersonalization is most marked when the client is most helpless, when the choice and arrangement of services are an exclusive prerogative of management.* In present day tax-supported service institutions, the client has a right as a citizen to obtain available services, but only if he is eligible. His "right" is only to services approved and financed by the state, and his eligibility is determined by the management's interpretation of the rules. The services themselves are underfinanced and frequently bare of what might be considered ordinary, everyday necessities. The client can exercise choice most easily when he has the financial or sociopolitical resources that allow him to obtain special privileges in the system.[6] The point is not that tax-supported institutions are inevitably or generically depersonalizing but that as they are *presently* constituted and financed they are likely to be. The generic variable underlying depersonalization is the status of the client: he is unable to choose and manage significant elements of his destiny.

Here is where the mental hospital, even when private, is relevant, for while there are differences in amenities and while relatives who are paying the bills exercise more leverage in private than public hospitals, depersonalization nonetheless occurs. The client may be made helpless in many ways, of which one of the most important in our day is being defined as socially and intellectually incompetent by virtue of mental illness or senility.[7] When his fundamental capacity to reason about reality is impugned, the patient becomes a ward of the service organization, public or private, and so becomes dependent upon the institution's choices made on his behalf.

But the main thrust of most analyses is not to deplore the patient's helplessness as much as to deplore the unprofessional character of the decisions that are being made on the patient's behalf. The idea is that even if patients are stripped of their ordinary freedom of choice, when managerial prerogatives of choice for the patient are exercised on a professional rather than lay basis, the patient will be considerably better off. From Belknap through Dunham and Weinberg to Strauss and his associates[8] (not to speak of a whole tradition of studies of "custodialism" in mental hospitals), attention is paid primarily to the fact that nonprofessional or unprofessionalized workers are largely responsible for the care of state mental hospital patients. As Strauss and his associates have demonstrated, the issue is not really the lack of a therapeutic orientation among those nonprofessional workers so much as the lack of a professionally approved orientation. If only there were more genuine psychiatrists dealing with patients, the argument runs, things would be so much better for them.

This rather simple argument has been extended much further. Great impetus was given to the idea that there can be an organization that is wholly therapeutic in character, without significant "pathologies" in the form of depersonalizing bureaucracy, by Stanton and Schwartz's study, reported in 1954.[9] The study's most celebrated findings (not fully borne out by later investigators) were that psychiatric symptomatology and at least the short-term progress of the patient in the small private hospital were related to the disagreements and tensions among staff members—related, in fact, to the total complex of relationships that makes up an organization as a whole. The idea was that individual psychotherapy carried out with the patient each day for an hour in the privacy of the consulting room, insulated from life on the ward, was no more and perhaps even less "therapeutic" than the other hours of the day spent in interaction with semiprofessional and nonprofessional personnel during the round of life on the ward. The rather more pallid and scattered study of Caudill[10] and a succession of minor reports have reinforced the general, even if not detailed, validity of the observation.

The Utopian Hospital

The outcome of the observation was the notion that the whole organization must be administered as a therapeutic activity and that everyone, professional and nonprofessional, must work together in order to be able to provide the proper milieu.[11] The whole complement of institutional personnel must become a team, undivided by status distinctions and "blocked communication," to create a therapeutic milieu. The patients themselves must be drawn into creating such a milieu and also serve as members of the team. This ideology, closely akin to some in industrial sociology, is essentially utopian, oriented toward blurring and even dissolving such elementary axes of rational organization as hierarchy and functional or task differentiation. Indeed, it is closely connected with utopian thought of the past and with latter-day nonmedical utopias.

Rubenstein and Lasswell's book offers us an interesting commentary on the plight of the utopian therapeutic community.[12] In 1951 and 1952 Caudill studied a mental hospital in which he noted a "caste" system among the staff in which physicians were authoritarian and the barriers between physician, nurse, and aide high and impermeable. In staff conferences participation was hierarchical. Without free and open communication among all staff members, much of what the patient did or said was misunderstood and mismanaged. Rubenstein and Lasswell describe how that same hospital began to move toward becoming a more "democratic" institution in subsequent years. In 1956 patients began attending staff meetings, and by 1960 patient–staff meetings were being held three times a week. As Rubenstein and Lasswell described it, nurses and residents were encouraged to take more active roles in therapy and patients themselves were encouraged to assume responsibility for managing the hospital as well as their own wards.

There were definite moves toward wider participation in administration and therapy but, as the authors noted with some sadness, the basic structure remained authoritarian. Residents and nurses were uncomfortable in their new roles and the senior medical staff would not allow the patients to assume very much responsibility for their own affairs. A totally equalitarian community of patients and staff seemed not to be viable. Indeed, it may be argued that by its nature a hospital cannot be a community in which each person exercises to the full his individual qualities, for it is neither self-sufficient enough to be able to violate the expectations of the society surrounding it nor able to overcome the constraints implicit in having a special mission or goal with special assumptions about the means of attaining it.

Unlike historical utopias, the hospital lacks some essential conditions of community and so can only be very loosely called a small society or a community. For one thing, even though power is exercised in the hospital just as it is exercised in the political community, the hospital is neither self-sufficient nor sovereign and so cannot make its own rules for the exercise of power by "citizens," including patients. Hospitals depend on the community outside for financial support quite apart from patient fees. Belknap and Steinle have shown that the relation of general hospitals to community leadership and financing is critical to the kind of hospital that can exist.[13] In their narrative, Stotland and Kobler demonstrate graphically how the arrogance, jealousy, and stupidity of a group of physicians and lay community leaders can destroy a hospital.[14]

The Position of Medicine in the Hospital

Hospitals, then, are not true, self-sufficient communities. They are communities only in the special fashion defined by Goffman: they are composed of those who live in and try to make a life of the hospital and those who live outside and carry on a job within. But there is an additional incompleteness in the American hospital that marks it off from virtually all other ordinary organizations. Except in many publicly supported hospitals, the prime members of the hospital staff are not employees, yet nonetheless they exercise extensive influence in the organization. The physicians responsible for the care given to the patients by other members of the staff are not themselves members of the staff in the usual sense of the term. This is a very unusual structural arrangement that has not been examined as closely as it deserves. It is as if all professors were self-employed tutors, sending individual pupils to universities where they can themselves administer some special training briefly, but most particularly where they can count on having their pupils trained specially by lesser personnel employed by the university rather than by the professor. The day-to-day service of the organization is supplied by people employed by the organization but supervised by self-employed entrepreneurs committed to their own personal practice and to the individual clients of that practice. The commitment of physicians, therefore, is qualitatively and quantitatively different from that of other workers in the American hospital.

In being dependent on the professional community outside for the voluntary supply of basic services its activities need, then, the American hospital is considerably less self-sufficient than the usual industrial or service organization, which hires its experts. The physician constitutes a continuous breach in the walls of the organization. As Stotland and Kobler's case study showed so graphically, the organization cannot even survive without the cooperative approval of those who are necessary but uncommitted by employment.[15]

The hospital "community," then, cannot do its work without the company of those who are not members and who, in Georgopoulos and Mann's summary of findings on ten hospitals, are "not too well integrated with the rest of the organization."[16] But why cannot doctors be dispensed with entirely, if they will not commit themselves wholly to the hospital? Obviously, quite apart from the fact that physicians often provide the customers needed by the hospital, they are needed because they are believed to have virtually exclusive possession of skill without which the essential tasks of the hospital cannot be performed adequately, without which the essential goals of the organization cannot be reached. And this points to what is perhaps the most profound problem of utopian equalitarianism—how individuality and equal participation in communal decisions can be maintained in the face of special competencies.

Differences in *power* can be leveled by agreement or force. Differences in bureaucratic *authority* can be dissolved by the abolition of office. But in the face of a given goal and belief that some special technique can gain the goal, *expertise* must be deferred to. The "authority" of expertise cannot go unheeded except at the expense of the goal. In this sense, I would argue that even if the hospital employed all its physicians (as is frequently the case in other nations) and had a most liberal endowment making it independent of the lay community, it could be either equalitarian or therapeutic but not both. So long as the goal of therapy is maintained and physicians are held to know how to achieve it, physicians will maintain a place of privilege and "authority" by virtue of their expertise quite independently of bureaucratic office, and patients will hold a place of subordination by virtue of their helplessness and ignorance. Similarly, when occupations are imputed skills of varying degrees of complexity and responsibility, differentiation will not only be horizontal, by task, but also hierarchical, by "responsibility," even if not by bureaucratic office.

In this sense, even if bureaucratic administration were to dissolve itself by some acid equalitarian zeal, its structure would be recreated by the hierarchical and functional needs of the application and coordination of special skills in a division of labor. The essentially unilateral, and therefore hierarchical, character of that division of labor was suggested by Georgopoulos and Mann's findings that "the extent to which the nursing staff understands the problems and needs of the medical staff, as seen by the latter, produces appreciably stronger relationships with each measure of patient care than the extent to which the medical staff understands the problems and needs of the nursing staff, as seen by the latter."[17]

Limiting Conditions of Hospital Care

What seems to be implied by this clutch of hospital studies, then, is that the essential attributes of formal organization (hierarchy and task differentiation) are no less requisite for the production of health services by "professionals" than for the production of material goods by "workers." In this sense, the interaction among the workers and between workers and clients must take on some of the impersonality and social distance characteristic of any rationalized organization of work. This is not to say that only formal relations are the rule. As decades of industrial studies have shown since the Western Electric study, there is no doubt at all that formal organization—"official" positions and rules—is only part of reality, and sometimes only an ideological or "mock" part at that. It is also true, however, that there is no doubt that in all the hospitals studied, stable limits to what can be negotiated are posed by position in both administrative and task structure. Insofar as that structure varies, so will the content and amount of negotiation.

One element of structure limiting interaction has already been alluded to in the distinctions between state and private, mental and general hospitals. Those distinctions bear on the position of the patient as a ward of the system versus the patient as a well-paying customer in a buyer's market and his position as a generally incompetent person versus that as a specifically incompetent or merely sick person. In the former, most extreme structural case, the patient is so little able to enter into negotiations as to be wholly depersonalized. At the other extreme, as in a luxurious rest home, the "patient" may dominate negotiations, being more a person than perhaps he deserves.[18]

In addition to the status of the patient, there is another factor that has very important influence on the content and amount of free interaction among patients and staff—the character of the task and the knowledge and technique actually available to accomplish it.[19] It seems no accident that the most marked variations in organization and in staff–patient and staff relations are to be found in mental rather than general hospitals. It is not in general hospitals that conditions can so easily vary from those of a concentration camp to those of a partially self-governing community. The organization of mental hospitals can vary so markedly because there is no clearly efficacious method of "curing" the mentally ill.[20] It seems that it is precisely the varied ideologies and technologies of psychiatry and its extraordinary therapeutic uncertainty that permitted the existence of the unstructured situations studied by Strauss and his associates. In the public mental hospital they studied, different wards were managed by physicians with different philosophies of treatment, and in the private institution, psychiatrists hospitalizing patients were of varied therapeutic persuasions and needs.

In contrast, a surgical ward such as the one studied by Coser is likely to vary considerably less in its organization, for its stable and frequently standardized therapeutic technology sets distinct limits on the degree of negotiation that can take place among the staff without interfering with the functional goals of the organization. Much the same regular and stable organization of authority and specialized task is likely to exist from one ward or hospital to another in such a case. The best of such organizations, in which one finds a smoothly operating team sustained by high morale, are nonetheless formal: good human relations must not mislead one into believing that members of the team are negotiating without limits. The task, the prerogatives of its practitioners, the equipment available to accomplish it, and administrative precedents all limit and constrain the behavior of the workers.

Contrast between psychiatric and surgical tasks leads us to the final point suggested by this review of hospital studies—that depersonalization even of an extreme sort occurs in instances that are not protested or deplored. The deprivation of consciousness, the complete immobilization and the literal objectification of the surgical patient is a case in point. This depersonalization is even more extreme than occurs in total institutions but it is acceptable nonetheless because it is seen to be a price worth paying for the benefits yielded. The depersonalization of the state mental hospital patient is an opposite case in point: while it may benefit the staff as an administrative convenience and the community outside by its contribution to the inexpensive custody of unwanted people, it is a price many believe is not worth paying for the benefits accruing to the patient. Similar evaluations of whether depersonalization is worth the benefit to the customer no doubt underlie some of the contemporary protests surrounding educational and welfare service institutions, both of which have "soft" technologies like those of mental hospitals.

The Problem of Professional Practices

In this context one may note that the most important task of the sociologist is not to document continuously and drearily the mere fact of depersonalization as a consequence of the rationalization of services. It is rather more valuable to evaluate the extent to which depersonalization is a necessary (or at worst mildly negative) consequence of the rationalization of a service sufficiently effective to make the price worth paying. For example, it is rather difficult to make much of an issue of Cartwright's findings that patients in teaching hospitals reported more impersonality than patients in nonteaching hospitals when she also cited findings showing that for selected diseases the mortality rates in teaching hospitals were lower than in nonteaching hospitals.[21]

Such crude calculations of cost are the least that may be done. The more subtle and complicated task lies in the analysis of the degree to which depersonalization is not related to the performance of an effective service at all, but is rather related to the worker's attempt to perform the service in ways that are in accord with his unscrutinized commonsense notions of what is theoretically or technically sound and compatible with his vested interests. The question is what elements in the organization and performance of work cannot be justified by the technical outcome of the work. Simple staff convenience of no benefit to the client is fairly easy to pick out if only because the worker himself is likely to label it such and defend it on nontechnical grounds. Much more complicated is the task of assessing the justification of the mass of practices comprising the worker's activity, most of which he justifies on technical grounds even though such grounds are not always demonstrable.

In the special type of service industry of which the hospital is one instance, the prime workers claim to be professionals and therefore claim immunity from evaluation by others. Furthermore, if their claim to professional status is honored by others, it is accompanied by a general belief in their expertise and concession of the authority of expertise. As noted earlier, the social establishment of expertise then permits the organization of services around its authority independently of purely administrative organization. However, it must be noted that expertise is merely imputed and may not in fact have a sound technical foundation.

Even in the corpus of such a scientifically based profession as medicine one finds a heart of solid skill surrounded by a large fatty mass of unexamined practices uncritically honored because of their association with the core skills. Some of that mass is composed of the social prerogatives claimed by the expert because of his professional status, though on occasion they may be justified technologically. Another portion of that mass is composed of the expert's commonsense world.[22]

The most important task of the sociologist in studying education and welfare as well as health factories is to dissect the fat from the muscle in the imputed skill of the professional service worker and to determine the consequence of each for what is done to the client, with what price. This task is so important because it is a moot question whether or not the rigidification of services is due to purely administrative bureaucratization. As I have tried to show, some aspects of organization stem specifically from the institutionalization of expertise. And since what is special about the health, education, and welfare factories is the great degree to which the prime worker is insulated from outside influence, from patient desires, and from inside, administrative influence by virtue of his professional status, the influence of expertise on depersonalization of services is particularly well worth emphasizing. In the new industrial sociology, the problem may lie less in management than in the worker.

Issues in Organizing Hospital Services

In all, this review points to the basic issue of the balance of influence in determining the way medical care is organized and presented in the hospital. Foremost is the problem of the balance between administrative and professional authority. By and large, in the general community hospital (which, unlike hospitals associated with medical schools, is representative of the domiciliary medical care to be found in the United States), administrative authority is rather weak and rudimentary and requires more support. The present need is for a variety of administrative mechanisms that can temper the arbitrary exercise of professional authority by the medical staff and institute procedures that give better assurance than exists at present that the quality of professional care is adequate. Some such mechanisms have already been required by the commissions that accredit hospitals for approved programs of postgraduate medical education (internships and residencies) and by federal, state, and even private organizations that, by virtue of insurance or some other obligation, pay some of the costs of hospitalization for individuals. In such cases, while review procedures are rightly carried out by the medical staff itself, they take place in the context of a set of requirements that contributes to the growing importance of a stable and influential administrative organization in the hospital, one that can act independently of the medical staff and press for policies of its own invention. It is, of course, possible that such an independent and influential administration can develop into a self-serving tyrannical management, but the prospects for such a disaster are quite slim as long as the professional staff remains the arbiter of the quality of its own work, which is, after all, the focus of the organization itself.

I would in fact argue that the administration or management of hospitals in the United States is not yet strong enough. It should be prepared to discriminate between the fatty tissue and the solid heart of medical work and to press for influence in trimming off medical jurisdiction over the fatty tissue. Much of what is called patient management, as distinct from the identification of illness, its cause, and its treatment, is not sustained or chosen by any systematic scientific knowledge, but rather by personal preference and experience and by occupational custom and folklore. As management, hospital administration should be prepared to take issue with medical dominance over that portion of medical work that influences the well-being and satisfaction of patients without at the same time having a technical or scientific rationale. Its weight, of course, should lie on the side of reducing professional control over patient choice and information to only that which can be justified by true medical knowledge and technique.

But in this it is too much to expect that enhanced administrative influence over patient care will always lead to benefits to the patient. Consonant with the stereotype of bureaucracy, management is naturally concerned first and foremost with the orderly and smooth running of organizational affairs and only then with the clientele. Unchecked, it too is likely to develop standard routines and procedures that reduce the institution's capacity to adjust to and properly serve patient and staff needs. Organized as it is, there is little immediate danger of the staff suffering greatly from such bureaucratization, but, if we take the understaffed state mental hospital as a case, there is much danger of the patient suffering. It seems appropriate that the patient himself, and his representatives, be equipped with their own leverage in the hospital to permit them to exercise influence independently of both medical staff and administration.

With the continued expansion of private and public hospital insurance, one socially crippling characteristic of patienthood—namely, being a "welfare" case who must be grateful for whatever he gets—is in the process of being eradicated. This is all to the good, but it is not enough, for welfare is not the only source of weakness in the patient's position. Particular diagnoses, such as senility, mental deficiency, and mental illness, impugn his capacity to choose what is in his own interest, as do states of fear and unconsciousness resulting from the acute and life-threatening illnesses taken to the hospital for management. Even if involuntary hospitalization and treatment were minimized, the social consequences of diagnosis remain for many conditions. Representatives of the patient do not, of course, always suffer from the same attack on their civil identities, so that where the patient cannot speak for himself, his representatives must be given more authority to negotiate on his behalf rather than to serve as mere visitors from the world outside who sign legal release forms. Indeed, governing boards of hospitals should be composed not merely of laymen vaguely described as community representatives but also of both past and present patients and of kin of past and present patients.

In spite of such devices, however, I believe that hospitals cannot fail to be much as they are today. Since they are devoted primarily to the treatment of cases sufficiently serious or dangerous to require domiciliary care, they require the kinds of management and treatment prerogatives that limit the activity and initiative of their clientele. Such management can be limited to only that which is necessary, but that which is necessary is nonetheless probably quite extensive. The only solution lies in restricting hospitalization (and the jurisdiction of hospitals) to the fewest possible conditions, finding instead a variety of ways of treating as many patients as possible on an ambulatory or home basis. I suspect that it is only insofar as hospitals in fact provide ambulatory services that they are amenable to radical change in the forces that shape their policies and procedures. And it is precisely ambulatory service, in and out of hospitals, that has come to require fairly far-reaching reorganization. Let us turn to the organization of ambulatory medical care now.

NOTES

1. For examples of such literature see M. T. McEachern, *Hospital Organization and Management* (Chicago: Physicians Record, 1957) and C. Wesley Eisele, ed., *The Medical Staff in the Modern Hospital* (New York: McGraw-Hill, 1967).
2. Erving Goffman, *Asylums, Essays on the Social Situation of Mental Patients and Other Inmates* (Garden City, N. Y.: Anchor Books, 1961).
3. Ivan Belknap, *Human Problems of a State Mental Hospital* (New York: McGraw-Hill, 1956) and H. Warren Dunham and S. Kirson Weinberg, *The Culture of the State Mental Hospital* (Detroit, Mich.: Wayne State University Press, 1960).
4. Peter Townsend, *The Last Refuge, A Survey of Residential Institutions and Homes for the Aged in England and Wales* (London: Routledge and Kegan Paul, 1962).
5. See Ann Cartwright, *Human Relations and Hospital Care* (London: Routledge and Kegan Paul, 1964) and Rose L. Coser, *Life in the Ward* (East Lansing: Michigan State University Press, 1962).
6. For example, English patients who can afford it may go to a private specialist in order to get a hospital bed quicker than they would from a National Health Service specialist, as reported in Cartwright, *Human Relations*.
7. See "The Moral Career of the Mental Patient" in Goffman, *Asylums*. See also the extensive analysis of illness in Part 3 of Eliot Freidson, *Profession of Medicine* (New York: Dodd-Mead, 1970).
8. Anselm Strauss, Leonard Schatzman, Rue Bucher, Danuta Ehrlich, and Melvin Sabshin, *Psychiatric Ideologies and Institutions* (New York: Free Press, 1964).
9. Alfred H. Stanton and Morris S. Schwartz, *The Mental Hospital, A Study of Institutional Participation in Psychiatric Illness and Treatment* (New York: Basic Books, 1954).
10. William Caudill, *The Psychiatric Hospital as a Small Society* (Cambridge, Mass.: Harvard University Press, 1958).

11. Ideologically connected with this movement is Maxwell Jones, *The Therapeutic Community, A New Treatment Method in Psychiatry* (New York: Basic Books, 1953).
12. Robert Rubenstein and Harold D. Lasswell, *The Sharing of Power in a Psychiatric Hospital* (New Haven, Conn.: Yale University Press, 1966).
13. Ivan Belknap and John G. Steinle, *The Community and Its Hospitals, A Comparative Analysis* (Syracuse, N. Y.: Syracuse University Press, 1963).
14. Ezra Stotland and Arthur L. Kobler, *Life and Death of a Mental Hospital* (Seattle: University of Washington Press, 1965).
15. As an occupational grouping in the state mental hospital, the psychiatric aides are so much better able to control treatment than anyone else simply because of the long-term commitment some of them have to the hospital, other occupational groups turning over more completely.
16. Basil S. Georgopoulos and Floyd C. Mann, *The Community General Hospital* (New York: Macmillan, 1962), p. 394.
17. *Ibid.*, p. 401.
18. For a very thorough examination of how the patient's treatment and management in the hospital are connected with his social class, see Raymond S. Duff and August B. Hollingshead, *Sickness and Society* (New York: Harper & Row, 1968).
19. For useful examination of the significance of the nature of the task to that of the organization, see Charles Perrow, "A Framework for the Comparative Analysis of Organizations," *American Sociological Review*, 32 (1967), 194–208.
20. For a more elaborate and stronger statement of this assessment see Charles Perrow, "Hospitals: Technology, Structure, and Goals," in James G. March, ed., *Handbook of Organizations* (Chicago: Rand-McNally, 1965), pp. 910–970.
21. Cartwright, *Human Relations*, p. 173.
22. Eliot Freidson, *Profession of Medicine*, Part 3.

7

Organizing Ambulatory Medical Care

For all its importance the hospital is not the major source of medical care. By far the greatest amount of medical service has always been provided to the public without hospitalization. And for that matter, some present-day movements stress the reduction of hospitalization. Most common in the past and the present is the service dispensed in the traditional doctor's office to which the patient goes when he has a complaint, where he is examined and treated, and from which he departs to return to his own home. On occasion, when the patient seems to be too sick to leave his home but not sick enough to be hospitalized without prior examination, the physician himself visits the home. All this constitutes ambulatory care.

Such care has significantly different characteristics and problems than the care of hospitalized patients, so even though some administrative unit of a hospital, such as an emergency room, a clinic, or an out-patient department, may on occasion provide routine ambulatory care, that unit nonetheless must be analyzed separately from the hospital proper as a distinctly different phenomenon. This is so because in the hospital there is no way of avoiding the problem of coordinating the provision of both technical and domiciliary services by a number of occupations. In the earliest hospitals as well as in those of today, physicians were not alone in providing care.[1] In the past others bathed the patient, fed him, and prayed with (or for) him; now others note his progress, give him medication, monitor the appliances on which his well-being depends, and the like. The hospital inevitably involves a division of labor among various occupations in the two tasks of caring for the patient and of providing for his domiciliary needs.

Unlike the hospital, ambulatory settings are characterized by a direct and simple relationship between client and consultant, with no other parties, neither "bureaucrats" nor "administrators," neither nurses nor technicians, involved. Under such circumstances there need be no separate "management," no bureaucracy, only the one worker who is himself both management and worker at the same time—in short, a "free professional." Of course, neither in the past, when there were dispensaries, free clinics, and charity clinics, nor in the present, with hospital emergency rooms, outpatient departments and clinics, and group practices, is ambulatory care always so simply organized as the private office.[2] But it can be and in many instances is. Such practice represents free self-directing work on the part of the physician, who is unfettered by hospital bureaucracy or other health occupations. Its problems may teach us something about the problems generic to the way physicians work. Therefore, I shall begin my examination of the problems involved in organizing ambulatory care by examining first this simple, individual office practice. Understanding it will facilitate the analysis of the more formal modes of organization that social policy is now emphasizing as a solution to the growing crisis of medical care in the United States.

The Market Organization of Individual Services

Superficially it would seem that individual office practice (or "solo" practice) is not an efficient or even methodical way of organizing care. However, it does constitute part of a methodical arrangement that could be considered rational and efficient if the goal of free individual patient choice of service is adopted. It is, of course, predicated on the freedom of clients to choose only among licensed medical practitioners, all other possibly competing healing occupations being at least in theory excluded from the market place in which the patient can exercise his choice. Furthermore, its essential and fundamental assumption is that every licensed medical practitioner has the same competence and ethical standards with no significant intrinsic differences among them. Such an assumption is absolutely necessary to justify allowing the layman freedom to choose the physician to treat him; only when all available physicians are equally competent does such freedom of choice by putatively uninformed laymen[3] pose no danger to their well-being.

Such standard competence, of course, need not be taken literally as equal capacity on the part of all physicians to diagnose and treat any condition or perform any procedure. Rather, it is competence to evaluate whether or not one *can* diagnose or treat a given condition or perform a given procedure as well as to determine who can do so and to be able to refer the patient to that person. Thus, in such a system of free patient choice it is assumed in theory that the physician chosen may be counted on either to manage the patient's complaint well or to refer him to someone who can manage it well. One has a picture of practitioners distributed through a community, each in his privately owned office, each freely chosen by a collection of patients, and each referring to appropriate others those cases he is not competent to manage.

A further degree of structure to the distribution is provided by those who limit their practice to special ailments, patients, or procedures, and who sometimes refuse to see patients who have not already been examined and referred by a physician of less limited or specialized practice. By virtue of the fact that lay as well as medical diagnosis of a complaint generally begins with considering it to be common and treating it routinely,[4] some practitioners deal mostly in the common everyday routine by which ailments are first defined and managed. Such primary practitioners are the first professional consultants in both lay and professional referral systems[5] or in the "hierarchy of resort,"[6] and by training they are often general practitioners, internists, and pediatricians. They are the ones who first see the patient and whose decision it is to treat him themselves or to refer him to another. In the free market setting of solo practice, that decision is, of course, a crucial test of the adequacy of the system. What pressures surround it?

To understand how the solo market operates, one must always bear in mind that it is dominated by the principle of individual free choice, with no self-conscious administrative organization imposed on it save that which determines the kind of practitioner who may legally offer services in the market place. Otherwise, every patient is free to seek services from whomever he will. Under such circumstances, it is inevitable that much choice will be based on considerations independent of the technical quality of the service. Just as consumption of the highly standardized mass products in today's market place seems to be based in part on such rational but marginal criteria as convenience and attractiveness in packaging rather than differences in quality of the product, so are patients inclined to choose their doctors on the basis of location, ethnicity, sex, personality, or bedside manner, more or less assuming competence until there is an occasion to make them feel otherwise.

In the solo market, the primary practitioner must possess the extrinsic characteristics that the lay community values or he will fail to attract enough patients to support himself. He must locate himself in a community with social prejudices to which he can conform. If he cannot do so, he must find another kind of practice. Lieberson's analysis of practice in Chicago suggests that when physicians of a given ethnic group exist in numbers too great to be supported by their own community, the surplus moves to downtown areas to serve the heterogeneous downtown population or to specialize and become colleague-dependent secondary practitioners.[7] While they are to a degree (which can be too easily exaggerated) liberated from conformity to lay prejudices, however, these secondary practitioners must instead conform to the prejudices of the primary practitioners who decide that their patients need specialized service.

The dependence of secondary practitioners on the referrals of primary practitioners for their trade means that a process of selection operates in referral relations just as much if not more than it operates in the formation of primary-care practices. A primary practitioner gradually builds up a stable lay clientele by a process of client selection; those who do not care for his ethnicity, background, location, hours, personality, manner, and therapeutic and diagnostic prejudices do not return after a trial visit. Over a period of time, those who may be counted on to visit him regularly have selected a physician who will have characteristics and practices that satisfy them. In some cases, of course, the physician will have adjusted himself to client therapeutic prejudices and in others he will have "educated" them to conform to his own taste. In neither case is it to his advantage to expose his clientele to a consultant or secondary practitioner who violates the prejudices which are the foundation of the relationship between client and referrer. He himself, therefore, by much the same process of trial and of negotiation of mutually acceptable procedures, tends to select the men to whom he refers by their compatibility with his and his clients' social and therapeutic preferences. Thus, just as the regular clientele of a given solo primary practice manifests a certain homogeneity, so does the collection of secondary practitioners with whom a given physician has regular referral relations. From the sparse evidence available, it appears that the homogeneity of membership in such referral circles tends to be a function of economic, social, and ethnic as well as medical compatibility.

Barriers to Free Choice of Ambulatory Services

The picture of the organization of ambulatory care I have just sketched is, of course, oversimple. The orderly sorting of patients and physicians into mutually agreeable, fairly homogeneous practices and referral networks cannot take place if there are barriers to choice created by factors other than individual social and medical taste. The fundamental barrier to choice that conditions the nature of the organization is, of course, that of medical licensing: individuals are free to choose only among practitioners who are licensed physicians and are not free to choose other kinds of healers.[8] This barrier is at the foundation of the whole system and is one that comparatively few people would criticize off-hand. But there is another barrier of major importance which, while generally recognized, has implications that are not often noted. I refer to the barriers created by a supply of physicians that is not sufficiently large and well-distributed to provide the patient with a broad set of alternatives among which to choose.

Notions of supply, demand, and need are even more problematic in the area of medical services than in areas that have traditionally preoccupied economists.[9] Like all needs, the interpretation of what is a medical need varies with historical, cultural, and professional conceptions of health; it is not a constant. Similarly, demand is not a constant, varying with conception of need as well as with conceptions of the role of the physician in serving need. One may evaluate supply only in the context of such variable needs and demands, but if one does, supply cannot be evaluated as a simple mechanical function of given needs and demands, for the unit of analysis by which one measures it is not self-evident. The unit is not really the physician but rather the varied services a physician may give. In this sense, simply the number of practicing M.D.s available to a population constitutes an extremely crude and possibly useless measure of supply, for if many patients demand preventive health services and few physicians are willing to give them, supply is limited to that few. The issue is also complicated by professional dominance, for in health as opposed to commercial affairs, the problem is not defined as meeting consumer demand no matter what it is. Rather, the profession insists on being the arbiter of whether or not a "need" really exists, whether or not the demand is appropriate to "true need," whether or not a service meets that need, and thus whether or not the supply of services is adequate. In medicine, much debate revolves around which services are "really" necessary and which are not.

Services are in fact juggled in the context of demand and supply. When individual physicians find that their case load or patient panel is becoming so large as to be difficult to manage with the time and energy they are willing or able to provide, they naturally attempt to reduce the absolute number of patients as well as the average time they devote to each one and the services they give. In solo practice in the United States, this is done in a variety of ways. One device is to raise fees in the hope of discouraging consultation for "trivial" complaints. A more common device is to reduce the convenience of services by requiring advance appointments rather than allowing people to drop in unexpectedly and by resisting if not always refusing to visit the sick patient in his home.[10] If the doctor is nonetheless confronted by a plethora of patients seeking services, the average amount of time assigned to dealing directly with individuals is reduced—commonly by having them examined or questioned first by some other person, such as a nurse or even a receptionist, and so made ready in advance for a purely functional examination on the part of the physician. This reduces the consumption of physician time and the absolute amount of physician interaction with the patient. Such reduction in the *quantity* of interaction and services generally results in a reduction in the content and *quality* of interaction in that the amount of time available for the casual social amenities so important in ordinary human relations is reduced.

In all this, given the desire both to reduce what is seen as an overheavy case load and to make its management easier, the practitioner becomes less flexible in the amount of time he is willing to give to negotiating with patients about the terms of the relationship. His services assume more of a take-it-or-leave-it character than is the case in other circumstances, and the patient must fit his anxieties, ignorance, and desires into the physician's brief encounter with rather less give-and-take than would exist in a market place where more choices are available to him. The physician is also less amenable to satisfying what he sees to be unnecessary or inappropriate demands—demands for house calls or for a walk-in emergency visit, to take the most common and least interesting cases, and also demands for vitamin injections, antibiotics, sedatives, tranquilizers, and other popular remedies. Furthermore, he is less inclined or able to spend time "educating" patients who make such demands.

While on occasion he may give them what they want out of sheer weariness, the physician is also inclined to manage especially demanding patients by merely getting rid of them or "dumping" them, suggesting that they go to some other doctor. In neither case is the physician likely to be able to adopt the time-consuming approach of "educating" patients or of attempting to determine the nature of the concerns or worries that may underlie the demand.[11] Patients in such a circumstance must either accommodate themselves to the requirements of the practice or get "dumped" into the market place to wander around looking for someone who will give them what they want or a service that will satisfy them some other way. But under the circumstances of short supply, the market place is so contracted that the shopper has rather few alternatives to choose from and may never find a satisfactory consultant.

Except perhaps in some urban neighborhoods where solo medical practice still remains somewhat competitive, the abbreviation of services has increasingly characterized the organization of ambulatory medical care in the United

States since World War II. While the medical market place is one in which the principle of free choice does exist as a possibility, it exists in reality for very few. A large segment, composed of the poor, the elderly, and the otherwise indigent, has for a long time been excluded from significant choice by virtue of inability or disinclination to pay the fees of the free medical market and has used other organized forms of ambulatory service. But by far the bulk of the population has participated in the system of organization I have just described. That system of individual practices, however, is becoming progressively more mechanized and rationalized and progressively less responsive to the tastes and desires of its lay clientele in spite of their being paying customers. And at the same time the system is becoming progressively more and more expensive. It must be emphasized that the growing crisis in the way ambulatory care is provided the average "paying" patient stems not only from the distinct and disproportionate recent rise in the cost of care for the individual consumer and his insuring organizations, public or otherwise, but also from its increasing inability to accommodate the human requirements of the individuals seeking care. Indeed, paradoxically enough, the character of solo practice in the private middle-class market place has more and more come to resemble the character of practice to be found in the organized settings that have traditionally provided ambulatory care to the indigent. Let us look at the nature of such settings.

Traditional Clinic Organization

The organization of care by solo practice in the United States is coming to resemble in many ways the care in clinics traditionally provided the indigent. There are indeed important differences between the two, the most important being the ecological convenience of the scattering of solo consulting rooms throughout middle-class communities, the physical amenities with which they are equipped, and the courteous if rather brisk demeanor of the practitioners toward their paying patients. In contrast, at the traditional charity clinic, free clinic, or hospital outpatient clinic, a number of practitioners are concentrated in a single place and their facilities are usually sparsely and unattractively furnished and at best routinely maintained. Courtesy is almost impractical because of the pressure of time on too few personnel, and it is discouraged as well by the status of the patients themselves, who, as welfare cases, are not treated as fully adult self-responsible persons.[12]

The absence of amenities is, to my mind, far more important than those who provide care within the clinic system are likely to admit; in teaching hospitals, for example, where those giving care are fairly well-trained or well-supervised, the staff is prone to assert that clinic or outpatient department or "service" patients receive technical care that is as good as if not better than that provided to "private" patients, except that it is presented without the "frills." It is apparently rarely considered that the frills constitute both recognition of the patients' dignity as human beings and an effective instrument for initiating a social relationship by which patients may be led to cooperate better with the needs of their treatment.

Be that as it may, clinic care has manifested exactly the same characteristics that have lain at the bottom of the growing criticism of the care provided to the ambulatory patient by physicians in private solo practice: inflexibility and brevity in the way service is provided, lack of concern for the personal convenience and desires of the patient, and a growing fragmentation of the services themselves. The latter is, of course, a partial function of the marked increase of specialized practices which virtually every commentator on the medical scene has noted and deplored at length and which need not be commented on again here.[13] It is also a function of a rational organization of work that relieves the private practitioner of the responsibility for being constantly available to his own patients whenever they need him. In order to have a satisfying private life, solo practitioners have developed arrangements whereby various colleagues take turns being on emergency duty for evening hours, weekends, and vacation periods. In such a circumstance the patient does not always see his "own" doctor. Without extremely careful communication, such a rotating system of coverage can contribute to the fragmentation of care.

While responsible for some of the present fragmentation, specialization does not inevitably lead to it; it is just that as the generalists have declined in number and intent, no device has arisen in solo practice to assure the coordination of the services of diverse specialists or some over-all responsibility for the patient as a whole. In theory these tasks are performed by the primary practitioner who refers his patients to specialists in solo practice, though in practice the patient is free to shop around himself among many kinds of specialists who do not require a referral from a responsible practitioner. In the traditional clinic there is often not even that primary referring agent to whom the patient returns after consultation with others. Furthermore, the traditional clinic is often staffed by practitioners who devote such a small proportion of their professional practice to the task that the patient's chance of seeing the same person on each visit, a single person who can assure continuity and responsibility for his care, is very poor indeed. Only the elaborate, cumulative medical record of the clinic (which is probably superior to that kept in the average solo practitioner's office) seems to serve as a counterbalance to truly dangerous fragmentation of attention and responsibility.

Underfinanced and understaffed as it is, the clinic stands largely as a model of the extremity to which medical care can go, an extremity toward which, for similar reasons, the solo method of organization is moving. In such an extremity care is fragmented into abbreviated service units among a number of practitioners, which provides no assurance that the continuity and coordination necessary to assure competent as well as personally satisfying care will be provided. The practitioners in the clinic work on terms (short hours, no housecalls, appointed consultation) which do not accommodate the personal convenience and habits of the clientele and which may not be sufficiently responsive to the knowledge or the emotional status of the clientele to assure either their cooperation or their satisfaction. But curiously enough, some of the organizing principles of clinic practice have been advanced as a solution to the problems of coordinating and financing medical care, problems that are increasing in solo practice.

Group Practice

As I have noted, the traditional ambulatory care available to the regularly employed, paying patient has been organized around the solo practitioner with his circle of self-selected patients and his links to consultants. Over time, the supply of services organized this way has failed to increase as rapidly as demand—partly because the absolute number of practicing physicians has not kept pace with the increase in population (let alone the population's rising expectations), partly because of the tendency of physicians everywhere in the world to wish to work in urban rather than rural areas, partly because of changes in the physician's own conception of the amount of time he wishes to reserve for leisure and his personal life, and partly because of the priorities physicians assign to the varied services asked of them. To cope with increased case loads, the solo physician has adopted a number of administrative tactics, all of which detract from the variety and the personal character of the services he gives and minimize the accommodation of those services to the patient seeking them. At the same time the continued growth of specialized knowledge and practice as well as of increasingly costly and intricate specialized equipment has made it more difficult to practice alone and use up-to-date consultant knowledge and equipment adequately.

Group practice is advanced as a possible solution to all these problems. Unlike the organization found in solo practice, which has been produced essentially unwittingly by the separate choices of individual patients and physicians in the medical market place, group and clinic practice are formal organizations consciously and deliberately organized to provide care. In such organizations a number of individuals practice medicine together. Group practice is usually said to be advantageous in a number of ways.[14] First, the fact that a number of physicians share the same facilities creates the possibility for economic advantages. Together, all can afford to have and use expensive equipment that would be out of their financial reach as individuals or that would be underutilized by one individual and therefore uneconomical for an individual practice. The sharing of common facilities is also likely to be economical in many ways, including clerical, paraprofessional, and office costs. Furthermore, group practice allows the individual to schedule his time commitments in such a way as to assure leisure untroubled by emergency calls. Finally, a major advantage of group practice lies in the technical quality of care it permits. Where men of different specialties work together in a group, consultation and coordination of care are thought to be facilitated. In addition, where men all work together in the same organization it is thought that they will stimulate each other to practice a higher standard of care than they might if each worked alone; in other words, each is "kept on his toes" by virtue of his continuous association with the others.

However, the advantages urged by the proponents of group practice do not exist in every form of group practice. The only characteristic common to all is, in varying degree, that of professionally determined rationalization of services. The process begun in solo practice whereby practice becomes less and less responsive to client demands by virtue of rationalization of professional convenience can, in fact, intensify in group practice. By bringing a number of men under one roof and into the same organization serving a local community, a more definite organization is in essence imposed on that which would have ordinarily existed in a looser form in solo practice. And since the practitioners all under one roof are likely to constitute a large proportion of the total number present in any single community (some medical groups including virtually all the practitioners in a town), their being formally joined together rather than being informally separate may operate to reduce the variety of choices and so the flexibility available to the layman. Decades of studies in industrial sociology have indicated that, in interaction in a formal organization, men are inclined to work out common, shared standards, social as well as technical, that order the level and direction of work effort. There is no reason to believe that physicians are immune to such processes, so that group practice may be seen to run the risk of enforcing standards that discourage soft-hearted concern for the patient's feelings, working longer-than-usual hours, and other forms of "rate-busting" which could more easily survive in solo practice.

Group practice is generally defined very loosely, as the following typical statement indicates: "Group medical practice is the application of medical services by three or more full-time physicians formally organized to provide medical care, consultation, diagnosis, and/or treatment through the joint use of equipment and personnel, and with the income from medical practice distributed in accordance with methods previously determined by members of the group."[15] Given the very general specifications in the definition, what assurance is to be found in them that the potential economies of group practice will indeed be used to increase capital investment in desirable technical equipment to improve services rather than used to increase profits by merely reducing the overhead of general operating costs per physician? What assurance is there that the economy of scale will be passed on to the consumer in the form of reduced fees rather than to the physician in the form of increased net income? As far as the public goes, there is no economic virtue to group practice unless the public benefits from it. Similarly, given the assertion of mere formal association among three or more men, without specification of the substance of that association, what assurance is there that the quality of medical care will be better than that in solo practice? Clearly, neither economy nor quality need follow from group practice defined so loosely. Without more concrete specifications, public support of group practice as defined is as likely to lead to further deterioration of health services as it is to lead to improvement. This can be seen when we examine one fairly common form of group practice found in the United States.[16]

This form of group practice is a simple aggregate of practitioners who have changed few of the habits they cultivated in solo practice. They work largely in their own offices on a fee-for-service basis, and their income more or less depends on the volume of their own work and the substance of their own billings. Instead of referring their patients outside their practice for consultation, however, they refer to a group colleague who, since he is part of the same practice and must live with the referrer, has rather less ground for independent action and opinion than he might otherwise have. The net result is a relative standardization of medical opinion and procedure, a reduction of diversity in practice.

Such standardization is likely to stem far more from the physicians who associate with each other continuously during their working hours than from the demands of the more transient patients who have no contract for services and who in any event are only occasionally in interaction with the members of the group. Sustained by formal group organization and continuous association, standardization is likely to be far more thoroughgoing than the common understandings joining referral networks in a solo community practice. And insofar as the group practice often embraces most if not all the practitioners in a given community, it markedly restricts the alternatives of choice available to the layman, thereby reducing his influence on the way in which services are presented to him as well as on the content of the services themselves.

In contrast, a much less common form of group practice in the United States frequently serves as a model for medical policymakers—the consumer-oriented prepaid service contract medical group in which physicians are often salaried or paid on a capitation basis. Under such a prepaid service plan, the choice of both physician and patient is limited. The physician supplies services only to those who are insured, and the insured can obtain services at no significant out-of-pocket cost only from physicians participating in the plan. Since there is putative free choice by physicians and patients in the community surrounding such medical groups (which are frequently islands in a sea of solo fee-for-service practice) and since that surrounding community is sometimes hostile, both patients and physicians may come to feel trapped by the plan and express resentment.[17] Furthermore, in such medical groups the necessity for the more elaborate records connected with service contract agreements, the existence of an outside insuring agency serving as the carrier of such agreements, and perhaps even the organization of the clientele into a definite group by such a contractual arrangement seem to make for rather more bureaucratic organization of work than is otherwise the case. While his autonomy as an individual may very well be reduced by such an arrangement,[18] the physician's capacity and motivation to join together with his colleagues to establish the social and technical standards of service to be presented to the clientele are certainly increased. The outcome seems to vary significantly when the consumer has a role to play in governing the service plan or medical group.[19]

Now clearly, some of this may seem to be all to the good. The standardization of procedure and opinion among working physicians and the minimization of therapeutic compromises due to patient pressure should yield some improvement in the *average* quality of work. But it could at the same time reduce all to that level, a standard that may not be absolutely high by more cosmopolitan or academic criteria. It can very well be the least common denominator of the local medical standards. Some device must assure higher standards than that. Furthermore, along with standardization of technical medical therapeutic practices in group practice is likely to go standardization of patient-management practices. The convenience and attractiveness of services to patients may become reduced to rigid standards enforced by the social processes familiar to students of industrial organization. The workers may come to present a united front to clients and superiors, using their own criteria of a fair day's work and of reasonable and dignified working conditions. Clearly, some device must assure that patient-management standards are properly responsive to patient needs. On both technical and humane levels, then, group practice can easily develop in such a way as to organize, standardize, and strengthen the reluctance of its members to accommodate themselves to the therapeutic prejudices and the human needs of its clientele. It could very well weaken the care provided to its clientele unless some mechanisms assure that the medical group recognizes the rights of the client and maintains high medical standards.

Defined simply as an association of cooperating physicians in a joint economic enterprise, then, group practice can vary quite markedly in consumer advantage from one medical group to another and can in fact operate in ways very much to the consumer's disadvantage. It can remove from the consumer's hands the last trace of leverage he possesses to gain responsiveness to his desires and needs. Whether or not variation is to the advantage of the consumer seems to depend upon a number of factors. Some, of course, involve the characteristics of the individuals who direct and work in the group, while others involve the administrative terms by which the group is organized.[20] Since personal characteristics of individuals are difficult to legislate (apart from establishing minimal formal standards for licensing and practice), however, the administrative characteristics underlying responsiveness to medical and consumer standards obviously represent those to which public policy must attend most carefully. Group practice is unlikely to constitute a solution to the problems grown so serious in solo practice unless it takes place in an organized environment that allows, encourages, and requires its members to strive to satisfy adequate standards. It seems appropriate to construct that environment from a variety of social and administrative devices, the most appropriate of which seem to be sufficiently flexible to accommodate individual needs but some of which must certainly be out-and-out bureaucratic. In the next and final chapter of this book I should like to suggest some of the methods by which ambulatory care in the United States can satisfy both technical and humane standards.

NOTES

1. For a brief history of the hospital, see George Rosen, "The Hospital: Historical Sociology of a Community Institution," in Eliot Freidson, ed., *The Hospital in Modern Society* (New York: Free Press, 1963), pp. 1–36.
2. For several reviews of the character of American medical practice, see Eliot Freidson, "The Organization of Medical Practice," in Howard Freeman et al., eds., *Handbook of Medical Sociology*, rev. ed. (Englewood Cliffs, N. J.: Prentice-Hall, 1970) and E. Richard Weinerman, "Research into the Organization of Medical Practice," *Milbank Memorial Fund Quarterly*, 44 (October 1966), Part 21, pp. 104–140.
3. There is some evidence that laymen are more capable of discrimination than professionals generally assume. See Arnold I. Kisch and Leo G. Reeder, "Client Evaluation of Physician Performance," *Journal of Health and Social Behavior*, 10 (1969), 51–58.
4. See, for example, Eliot Freidson, *Patients' Views of Medical Practice* (New York: Russell Sage Foundation, 1961).
5. *Ibid.*

6. Lola Romanucci Schwartz, "The Hierarchy of Resort in Curative Practices: The Admiralty Islands, Melanesia," *Journal of Health and Social Behavior*, 10 (1969), 201–209.
7. Stanley Lieberson, "Ethnic Groups and the Practice of Medicine," *American Sociological Review*, 23 (1958), 542–549.
8. Cf. Richard H. Shryock, *Medical Licensing in America, 1650–1965* (Baltimore, Md.: Johns Hopkins Press, 1967).
9. See, for example, Rashi Fein, *The Doctor Shortage: An Economic Diagnosis* (Washington, D. C.: The Brookings Institution, 1967).
10. For two examples of the limited material available about housecalls, see M. Clyne, *Night Calls, A Study in General Practice* (London: Travistock, 1961) and W. W. Forbes, "Lubrucationes: An Analysis of Two Hundred Eight Calls," *New England Journal of Medicine*, 253 (1955), 60.
11. For one psychiatric analysis of patient relations, see Michael Balint, *The Doctor, His Patient, and the Illness* (New York: International Universities Press, 1957).
12. In an interesting study, Ellis suggests that London physicians were forced to deal with "charity cases" by the competition posed by apothecaries. See Frank H. Ellis, "The Background of the London Dispensary," *Journal of the History of Medicine*, 20 (1965), 197–212.
13. See, for example, D. Rutstein, *The Coming Revolution in Medicine* (Cambridge: Massachusetts Institute of Technology Press, 1967).
14. For recent policy discussion about group practice, see "Promoting the Group Practice of Medicine," Public Health Service Publication No. 1750 (Washington, D. C.: U.S. Department of Health, Education, and Welfare, 1967).
15. This is the slightly modified version of the definition of the American Medical Association to be found in B. E. Balfe and M. E. McNamara, *Survey of Medical Groups in the U.S., 1965* (Chicago: American Medical Association, 1968), p. 2.
16. Underlying these characterizations is information from *ibid.* and from the materials reported in Eliot Freidson and Buford Rhea, "Physicians in Large Medical Groups: A Preliminary Report," in Kerr L. White, ed., *Medical Care Research* (Oxford: Pergamon Press, 1965) and as yet unreported findings from the Freidson and Rhea study.
17. The Freidson and Rhea study found marked association be-

tween consumer prepaid plans and physicians' feelings that patients were ungrateful.

18. Engel found that autonomy as she measured it was increased by moderate but not great bureaucratization. See Gloria V. Engel, "The Effect of Bureaucracy on the Professional Autonomy of Physicians," *Journal of Health and Social Behavior*, 10 (1969), 30–41.

19. See the findings in Jerome L. Schwartz, *Medical Plans and Health Care: Consumer Participation in Policy Making with a Special Section on Medicare* (Springfield, Ill.: Charles C Thomas, 1968).

20. *Ibid.*

8

Professional Dominance and the Reorganization of Medical Care

It might be thought that the aim of medical service is the provision to its consumers of care that is of the best possible technical quality. Such is not the whole case, however, not even for animals. They, after all, have their Society to protect them against cruelty. For human animals, perhaps, we can expect more than such a society to temper the way diagnostic and therapeutic techniques are applied. Medical service must be of the best possible technical quality, true, but it must also be of the most satisfying possible human quality. Whether it is true or false that humanly satisfying care has its own technically therapeutic value, it is nonetheless a moral necessity.

Medical care must, of course, be freely available to all independent of personal income. I regard that as an obvious requirement. But it is not enough, for though the future will almost certainly see the elimination of any significant financial barriers to medical care, if only that minimal reform took place with no others accompanying it, all patients, not merely that unhappy minority of the financially incapacitated in the present, would become welfare patients in the future. Medical care must constitute a personal service to human beings who have a right to the dignified status of adults who participate in determining what happens to them. In this chapter I shall try to suggest means of encouraging such care.

The Problem

While the beginning of this book addressed itself to specifying the character of the discipline of the sociology of medicine, it focused within that discipline on the smaller but more strategic question of the nature of the profession that creates, teaches, and applies the knowledge and skill of medicine. In the course of exposition the analysis has become narrower and narrower, moving from a very broad view of the health division of labor and the place of the medical profession in it to the medical profession itself and only finally to the concrete institutions that provide medical care. Nonetheless, even in the latter case I have tried to stress general analytical variables more than the detailed facts of today that will have changed tomorrow. And in all cases, consonant with the "structural" or "environmental" approach I specified at the outset of this book, I have stressed the consequences of the organized setting for the way medical work is carried out, as well as the consequences of the special institutionalized status or position of a dominant profession like medicine. In the course of my analysis I could not help but compare the character of the profession's special status and authority with that of the bureaucrat, manager, or administrator.

The outcome of that comparison of professional and bureaucrat emerges as one of the central points of this book, for while it is virtually universally agreed that bureaucratization creates the possibility (all too often realized) for the exercise of official authority in a way that reduces human clients to mere passive objects and ciphers lacking the right to participate in the process of shaping the service they get and to gain a reasonable amount of satisfaction of their own individual needs, it is almost as universally assumed that professionalization does not pose such problematic possibilities. I have pointed out, however, that professional authority is more similar to bureaucratic authority than is generally recognized and that the outcome of the use of such authority by a dominant profession like medicine is more similar to the "pathologies" of bureaucracy than is generally realized. Indeed, unlike professions, which have at the very best a vague set of usages and norms specifying the human rights of patients, rational–legal bureaucracies do have by their very nature formal rules and procedures that specify at once rights and modes of appeal to such rights. Without implying that bureaucratic procedures work out any more ideally in practice than do professional norms, I concluded that the rights of the patient and even the range and quality of the care given to him would be better protected if the autonomy and dominance of professional authority were checked and balanced by the pressure of an independent, extraprofessional administrative authority. But since administration has its own needs independent of and sometimes conflicting with those of the client and the professional, it too requires tempering. While the strengthening of administrative influence over the way professional work is performed is important, the strengthening of the influence of the client on both is perhaps more important.

The client, after all, has his own perspective on his service, a perspective that is not, like that of those who serve him, compromised by additional commitment to the provision or administration of service. Indeed, I should say that if the health services of the future are to be organized more economically, fairly, and "rationally" than they have been in the past, the only thing that can save them from accelerating the emerging crisis in the human quality of their care is the concomitant strengthening of the circumstances that permit the patient to have direct impact on the care he receives as an individual. Legislative or "community" representation is too gross and insensitive, too slow-moving and indirect to be sufficient; as I shall note shortly in more detail, the organization of patients into direct, local confrontation groups is likely to do more damage than good. The problem is to develop a medical service organization that creates an environment that stimulates both good technical care and care that is responsive to the immediate human needs of the patient.

Goals of Medical Service

I take it as axiomatic that concrete modes of organizing health or any other human services should be quite varied in content so as to be adjusted to varied management and patient problems. In order to avoid the imposition of a destructively rigid and meticulous scheme on such varied circumstances, it is essential that guiding assumptions be emphasized over specific procedural or organizational mechanisms. The danger of dogmatic commitment to specific solutions is very great in dealing with such issues as the mode of financing the costs of medical care, the mode of paying the doctor, and the mode of organizing care, for some solutions have emerged as ideological tokens in a historical struggle between state and profession. Furthermore, vested interests have grown up around the several alternatives contemplated—the private insurance industry and trade unions, for example. Any alternative actually chosen is in the nature of the case bound to be the political product of a compromise of varied interests and ideologies which should be recognized frankly as such. In the light of those realities, no scheme for the future is likely to be created and actually instituted *de novo*. While there are very good economic and administrative reasons for recommending a scheme based on salaried group practice financed by compulsory, federally administered health insurance, political realities may actually lead to financing fee-for-service solo practice with public insurance funds administered by private carriers. Without assuming that an ideal scheme will ever emerge, are there any conditions under which even an undesirable mode of organizing health services may be led to provide good, even if expensive care? This is the question I wish to answer now by outlining what I regard as essential principles for obtaining good care no matter what may be the concrete ways of organizing practice and administering its financing. The clearer the guiding principles and the more pragmatic the view of the mechanisms by which those principles can be realized, the better the practical chance of developing a reasonably good system of health care in a democratic society that must be responsive to varied interests and pressures.

It may well be that writers on medical policy indulge in the greatest amount of wishful thinking when they assess the way various alternatives advance the basic goals of reducing the burden of the cost of care and improving the quality of care. There is virtually no reliable systematic evidence on the quality of patient care available to justify the preference for solo practice asserted so forcefully by organized medicine in the United States. Similarly, while there is some, there is hardly enough systematic, empirical evidence to sustain the preference for group practice asserted by present-day medical policy makers. Virtually all the literature available on the organization of medical practice relies not on systematic data collection but on special pleading, extremely limited administrative records, and inevitably biased reflections by practitioners or medical administrators on their personal experience with one or another kind of practice.[1] Study of medical practice by outsiders free to collect what data they wish is extremely rare, so that choice among types of practice is today made more on the basis of personal or ideological preference than on the basis of reliable information. In the light of this deficiency, it becomes all the more important that the logic underlying choice between alternatives be stated clearly and forcefully, for it, not good evidence, is all we have to guide choice in a time when choice cannot be put off any longer.

What general goals are reasonable? The first, to which probably everyone will subscribe, is that the average care provided by the average practitioner to the average patient must be of the highest possible technical quality. A second is that all the care that falls below average should never fall below the level of the acceptable. A third goal is that below-average care, even if medically acceptable, should never be tolerated if it is distributed systematically rather than randomly, that is, if it is prevalent mainly in services to special groups like the poor, the elderly, the mentally ill, or the uneducated. Finally, and not least important, medical care should be humanly attractive enough to encourage its ultilization and satisfy its clientele.

These assumptions, however, are almost pious in their generality and provide only the vaguest of guides for social policy. Many will agree with them but disagree on how they may be realized in a concrete plan for reorganizing medical services. What is needed in addition are principles addressed to the question of organization itself, based on the evidence available about the way medical care systems function. A great deal of my analysis in the past chapters has been addressed precisely to such evidence and allows rather more direct formulation of principles to guide the reorganization of the procedures by which medical care may be given. I suggest five such principles here.

Principles for Reorganizing Medical Care

Above all, qualifying all else, is my contention that both past and present evidence and experience do not support the justice of the profession's claim for autonomy in organizing the way it presents care.[2] Thus, we cannot rely solely on the profession and its own system of self-regulation to provide a responsible system of care. Second, it should be clear that some kind of legal, administrative, or bureaucratic system is needed to provide an organized set of requirements that stimulates the profession to provide responsible care and the political and economic support to sustain such care. Third, I might point out that since bureaucratic procedures contain their own incipient pathologies, it is important that they be limited, if possible, to indirect and parsimonious mechanisms open enough to allow a great deal of variety and flexibility in how they meet the standards they lay down. Fourth, it is absolutely essential to the provision of humanly satisfying, not merely technically adequate, care that the patient be in a position of sufficient independence to be able to exercise choice and have a voice in the organization, presentation, and substance of the care he gets. Fifth, since organized confrontation and formal contractual agreements produce their own forms of rigidity and destructiveness, it is important that we emphasize methods by which *individual* rather than organized patients are able to exercise effective influence, for when varied individuals are able to exercise influence, the system must keep itself somewhat flexible in order to be accommodating, and cannot create any rigid method of standardizing services.

These principles for organization may also, like the assumption specifying goals and criteria, seem extremely vague, but I believe that they are nonetheless sufficient to imagine concrete ways by which the aims of the system may be advanced, ways that establish an organized environment within which the average physician, administrator, and patient are encouraged to play their roles well rather than ways that presuppose that by some unlikely process of professional and patient education the average individual will be so well molded as to be able to perform adequately independently of his environment. Let me suggest some concrete possibilities to indicate how those principles can guide the construction of various environments in which ordinary men are encouraged to make the most of their capacities.

The Financial Foundation of Medical Care

Much controversy revolves around the ways the cost of medical care is to be financed and how the money available is to be paid. Almost everyone seems to agree that the insurance principle should guide the financing of care so that the burden is not borne solely by the sick at the time of their need for care. In the United States organized medicine generally seems to prefer that private rather than public agencies serve as the carriers of such insurance. The issues for policy are whether private carriers would cost more money than public carriers and if so, whether that extra cost would nonetheless be worth paying and whether such private carriers would be at once accountable to the public and active in ensuring that the medical care they pay for is adequate. A private carrier that is actively concerned with the quality of care it insures is not an impossibility.[3] The type of carrier, therefore, may be judged on standards of cost and responsibility, independently of political ideology about the virtue of public versus private organizations.

Perhaps more complicated than the issue of carrier is the question of how the insurance funds are to be paid to those who provide care to the sick.[4] The weight of governmental policy opinion generally favors a service plan in which the patient is guaranteed all the services he needs without a fee for each service, for by this means the sick are not specially taxed because of their sickness. Similarly, such opinion favors a capitation or salary plan whereby the physician is paid by the insurer to provide all needed services to those who fall sick in a given population. In contrast, the opinion of organized medicine generally favors an indemnity plan whereby the patient is compensated for some costs incurred in seeking care from physicians to whom he himself directly pays a fee for each service. The former is easier to administer and control financially while the latter grants the practitioner considerably greater financial and administrative latitude (including the opportunity to charge a fee greater than the insurance indemnity compensation to the patient). The former is probably a less expensive method of paying for care than the latter.

Both methods have disadvantages for assuring the quality of the care provided, however. Since a salary or a capitation scheme of paying the doctor constitutes payment for care in general rather than for specific services, it removes direct financial incentives to provide individual services. Thus, it may operate to discourage the provision of needed services and perhaps encourage overprescribing as a quick and simple way of getting rid of demanding patients. The fee-for-service system, however, may encourage the provision of "unnecessary" services in the form of many return visits as well as much surgery and other procedures for which a fee may be charged, for the more individual services the physician gives, the more his income increases. Obviously, each alternative, if adopted, must be accompanied by its own administrative mechanisms specifically designed to counteract the disadvantageous tendencies to which it is prone.

But apart from medical, administrative, and economic standards of the technical quality and quantity of care, there are also human standards. I do not believe that these may be sustained adequately solely by professional and bureaucratic services designed to "protect" the patient. Only a system that provides the individual patient himself with the opportunities and resources to exercise his own choice of practitioner and service is likely to sustain such human standards. In evaluating that problem in the light of paying the physician, it seems to me that the most flexible and direct method of supplying individual patients with such choice as individuals (rather than as members of some organized group negotiating contracts) is the fee-for-service method. By the nature of the method, one patient's decision to use a physician's services is directly and immediately translated into a financial benefit to the practitioner chosen. This does not mean that a capitation or salary basis of payment cannot be set up in a way that allows fairly flexible patient choice, but only that fee-for-service provides the most direct and *immediately conse-*

quential means of doing so. Furthermore, it is most easily refined as a flexible method of control by the insurer or the insured: they may refuse to pay a fee for any single unacceptable service rendered, and are thereby able to exert sanctions over every *single* unacceptable action on the part of the practitioner. Should such acts be numerous, the consequences to the practitioner would be cumulative. Should they be few and scattered in the course of a normal practice, the consequences would be minor. Such a detailed and flexible response to practitioner deviance is not so easily made where salary or capitation fees are involved, for in that case each single instance of unacceptable service cannot be dealt with easily as it happens: the service must be extremely and continuously bad before one can do something so drastic as reduce or eliminate salary or capitation fee.

It is important, however, to recognize that none of the methods of paying the doctor, including fee-for-service, will be able to encourage significant responsiveness to patient choice if the available services and practitioners are so few in number and variety as to present no viable alternatives for choice and differential reward. As I have noted in the last chapter, solo fee-for-service practice in the United States today provides too few practitioners and practitioner services to permit very much significant choice to the consumer or to be significantly responsive to consumer desires. No matter how the doctor is paid, the circumstances of practice must be such as to require substantial competition of some kind among medical care institutions and practitioners for patients. Without such competition there is little likelihood that services will be responsive to the human needs of the clientele rather than only to those needs recognized by profession and administration. When competition for clients is lacking and when both practitioner and client are bound together by a long-term prepaid service contract, there is a very real danger that one or the other or both will feel hopelessly captive and that the human if not the technical quality of service will suffer correspondingly. However services may be financed, some competition must be built into the system.

Competition in Medical Care

It is clear that the social organization of competition is as important as the financial mechanisms of insuring and paying for medical care, and should in fact vary independently of them. Solo practice, for example, need not be uninsured, nor need it be fee-for-service, as the present National Health Service in Great Britain shows. Group practice too need not be founded on some prepaid insurance scheme, nor need its practitioners be salaried or paid on a capitation basis, as the majority of American medical groups testifies. While methods of financing the cost of care and of paying the doctor constitute importance sources of incentive and stimulus for performing certain desirable services, the social organization of care can provide additional incentives and stimuli. Most often mentioned in this context is the position of the solitary practitioner who, lacking continuous interaction with colleagues, is not exposed to important sources of stimulation that may keep his technical work up to date. But by the same token, the solitary practitioner in a competitive milieu is not in a position to be organized by his colleagues to present a common front to patients seeking services, and so may be more flexible in meeting their human even if not their technical needs.

I think that there is enough evidence available from the study of formal organizations to allow us to take as axiomatic the premise that when men work together in the same place, on the same terms, and with common work problems, they will develop a set of standards and procedures by which to judge and manage those problems, and they will discourage deviation from those standards.[5] In medicine some kinds of colleague deviance may be labeled incompetence, carelessness, sloppiness, or lack of conscientiousness. Other kinds may be labeled spoiling the patient, overpermissiveness, or unethicality. Merely the fact of participating together in the same organized setting provides no assurance that the actual standards colleagues do agree upon and enforce will be either technically or socially adequate: the only assurance is that there will be standards of some kind and that they are likely to be narrower and better enforced than if the same men were scattered through a variety of settings, competitive or otherwise. All else being equal, I would guess that technical standards would on the average be higher and the range of variation narrower in an organized work group, while social standards would on the average be lower. What must also be added to the virtues of solo practice is its spatial distribution: it is likely to provide primary even if not special, secondary services in more convenient locations than can organizational practice.

If my premise about the potential dysfunctions of organizational practice is true—and much more evidence supports than contradicts it—then it follows that considerable caution must be exercised in developing new forms of medical care organization. The ideal picture of solo practice advanced by organized medicine should not be rejected out of hand merely because it does not reflect reality (or because it is advanced by organized medicine): it represents a very flexible method of providing primary care that can, under some circumstances, be very satisfying to both physicians and patients. Furthermore, much of its technically undesirable isolation may be counteracted without too much difficulty by the telecommunications technology that already exists, not to speak of such devices as the videophone which are on the near horizon. And since the communication of information in our society is far easier and cheaper than the transportation of human beings, there may be very practical advantages for the patient in avoiding the ingathering of physicians into centers to which every patient must always go for his care, an ingathering that occurs at the same time as both public and private transportation becomes increasingly difficult. Cost aside—and cost is in any case so slippery a notion that few have claimed that the savings to be gained by practice in an organized setting will actually reduce the cost rather than merely expand the scope of care—solo practice remains a viable alternative for the provision of care of a high technical and social quality *as long as a careful administrative framework is built around it to assure such quality*. Given the fact that many physicians seem to prefer such solo practice[6] it does not seem wise to ignore either those of its potentialities that should be encouraged or those that should in some way be discouraged.

The Administrative Organization of Medical Care

I have already pointed out the evidence for the belief that professionals are not likely to maintain a high standard of both technical and personal care when left to their own devices. Their work environment must be such as to stimulate them to establish and maintain high standards. Assuming that payment for care will in most if not all cases in the future ultimately come from some insuring organization, it is essential that payment be in some way contingent on meeting the requirement of high standards. Assuming that the least expendable product is care that minimizes the killing and disabling of patients and maximizes the promptness of relief from and cure of their ailments, the first and most indispensable requirement is assurance of adequate supervision and review of the quality of medical work. The mere association of colleagues does *not* provide such assurance: like long-married couples and workers everywhere, colleagues become tolerant and protective of each other, particularly when precedents threatening to accustomed routines are demanded by obstreperous patients or raised by malpractice suits or any other outside agents or events. Furthermore, professional etiquette itself discourages observing and criticizing one's colleague's work. Only the requirement of *formal periodic internal review* of the quality of their work is likely to stimulate practitioners to look closely at what each is doing and to evaluate work by some systematic self-conscious standard. Such review makes the work of each observable to the other in spite of the barriers to visibility erected by etiquette and the private nature of medical consultation itself, and constitutes self-conscious examination of work that counteracts the fluid nature of informal processes of control.

However, internal review in itself is not enough, for as I have already noted, the tendency is for practitioners to associate with those who share their standards, thus producing separate, homogeneous circles of practitioners of varied standards—high and low, realistic and academic—each circle insulated from the regular observation and evaluation of the other. Formal review within a practicing collectivity merely encourages further compliance of individuals with the standards of that collectivity; it does not assure that the standards themselves will be of an absolutely high quality. What is necessary to assure such absolutely high quality is additional review by outsiders who represent the highest possible standards of the profession as a whole. Only the requirements of a *formal, periodic, outside professional review* can provide the counterlever to the tendency for the development of self-sustaining parochial standards in varied practice settings. And such outside review would also sustain the practitioner in resisting those demands of his local clientele that are technically undesirable.

Outside review should, of course, be concerned first of all with such essentially mechanical issues as the method used by the local circle of practitioners in its own required internal review, the completeness of medical records, and the formal qualifications of the physicians involved for the work they perform. Equally important, though, is assessment of the referral and consultation patterns to be found in the local circle, the methods by which care is coordinated or fragmented, and, not least of all, the propriety, skill, and decency of the practitioner's manner of dealing with his patients. In order to protect patients' rights and to sustain the social quality of care, outside reviewers should assume that consultation room manner is as important a consideration of good professional care as diagnostic perspicacity. Perhaps randomly drawn patients could be both examined and interviewed about their care by such a visiting review, thereby serving as an additional source of information and perspective from which to evaluate the quality of performance of the physicians being evaluated.

Given such information, outside review can operate like accreditation committees for hospitals and educational institutions by providing the foundation for periodic reconsideration of the formal status of the community or group of practitioners. Individuals, circles, or groups can, on the basis of review, be excluded from support or put on probation by public or insurance funds if they fail to meet standards. They can have their approval or accreditation renewed after demonstrating improvement, or they might even be able to gain a special meritorious position whereby they are eligible for greater support than those who are merely acceptable—support in the form of higher fees, salaries, or subsidies.

In considering the requirements of both internal and outside review of records and practice, it is of critical importance to be aware that they can be applied as well and as effectively to men in solo practice. There is nothing to prevent solo practitioners in the community from constituting their own "internal" review committees. Nor is there anything in the nature of solo practice (save its ideology of rugged individualism) to prevent visits from outside review committees. The requirement of internal review is likely to encourage interaction among solo practitioners and discourage isolation, and if they truly performed the review required of them, their interaction would have to revolve around the issue of standards of medical care. The requirement of outside review and evaluation may be expected to function in both solo and group practice to prevent the standards of the local community practitioner from settling down into a too comfortable and progressively antiquated routine.

The Role of the Client in Medical Services

Important as the administrative requirement of professional review is for sustaining the quality of medical care, it is not enough. It is not enough precisely because it is administratively initiated and professionally implemented. It protects what insurance carriers, administrators, and professionals see as the best interests of the patient, but it may very well exclude protection of what patients themselves feel are their interests. While patients' conceptions of their interests may be as mistaken as are administrative and professional conceptions, and may in fact be self-damaging, they should be both expressed and emphasized independently of administration and profession. There is no proper surrogate, no substitute for the direct expression of his interests and needs by the patient himself.

Most discussions of the patient's role assume that the good intentions of the professional practitioner are enough to protect the patient. Such good intentions do indeed protect the patient to some degree, but not sufficiently to constitute adequate protection. Some discussions seek such protection by stressing the importance of patient or consumer representation on governing boards of health insurance plans, hospitals, clinics, medical groups, and, I must add if we take solo practice into account as a possibility, local community medical boards. A small number press for the organization of patients into pressure or even confrontation groups. Let us look at each of these three.

I have already indicated that I believe good intentions on the part of administration and profession cannot overcome their inevitable bias in perspective. Each perspective has its own legitimate interest that prevents it from adequate sensitivity to the perspective of the patient. Second, I may say that I certainly believe that consumer representation on formal governing boards is necessary and useful, but the problems of maintaining the integrity of such representation in the face of cooptation by other members and the "professionalization" of the consumer representatives themselves lead me to believe that such representation is not enough and may in fact on occasion constitute a hoax. The third device, mobilization of patients themselves into organized action groups, is, to my mind, a last resort, appropriate only when all other devices have failed and when services remain nonetheless rigidly unresponsive to patient needs. When patients are organized into such groups, issues become undesirably stereotyped and negotiation takes place in terms that are not likely to serve the mutual benefit of all parties. It would be a tragedy if medical (and, for that matter, educational and welfare) services were so deeply resistant to accommodation of client needs that confrontation politics became the rule of the day. I think it can be avoided by a properly designed system of care.

A properly designed system does not require such group mobilization because it is sufficiently flexible and well-intentioned to respond to *individual* patient needs and because individual needs can be expressed in a way that has an impact on the system. Such a system is likely to be created and maintained when it is organized around the structural devices that encourage flexibility and self-expression. The basic characteristic of such a system must be its emphasis on the individual patient's capacity and right to make significant choices among a variety of elements in his care. Such an emphasis is not possible in a fully "administered," uniform system built around professional and administrative standards alone. Absolute patient dominance is not, of course, the alternative I am suggesting. Rather, I suggest an alternative that permits effective, countervailing pressure from the patient to temper professional and administrative modes of providing service by allowing the patient to choose among alternatives. Such a system should allow patient choice and, by having competition among practices and services built into it, should present a setting in which choice has consequences of real advantage to those chosen. Advantages to the provider of service can come from a variety of concrete consequences of choice, including the material rewards of additional or higher fees, capitation sums, salaries or merit awards, and the reward of honor to be found in rank, citation, or whatever. Always assuming that both internal and external professional review are present to sustain sound medical standards and thus to prevent individual and organized practices from competing for patient favor by merely giving the patient whatever he wants (with whatever medical risks and consequences), a system involving some kind of competition for patient choice is essential.

The best and likely most flexible and progressive of the possible ways of organizing the system is also the most expensive, since it deliberately encourages some degree of overlap and duplication of services and resources by requiring that there be alternative practices to choose from in the local community or neighborhood—two neighborhood health centers or medical groups for each neighborhood, for example, not one, and/or more solo practices than strictly necessary—but all subsidized by insurance funds so that a basic income is assured any creditable practice no matter what its popularity. Such a situation resembles that of earlier days, when the supply of physicians per capita was greater and the demand for services lower and more restricted. It is different in being supervised professionally and in being given minimal economic security. This system is likely to be too expensive to be espoused by policy makers, however. By design or more likely by default, greater parsimony and "rationality" are likely to characterize the system of the future. Nonetheless, whatever the system becomes, the units within it—whether solo or group practitioners or individual units organizing service within health centers or medical groups—must in some way be competitive with one another. In this way the components of the system will be encouraged to experiment with new ways of providing service, to serve the individual patient more as he wishes in the light of professional standards, and to devote itself to teaching and persuading the patient of the value of professional recommendations.[7] In all cases, there would be less reliance on professional and administrative authority and more on the authority of honest expertise. Circumstances should oblige practitioners to keep the patient as fully informed about his treatment as possible, to give truly informed consent and cooperation, and to be willing to allow the patient to choose among the diagnostic and treatment options that exist and that are recognized as preferences, opinions, and schools among professionals themselves.

How can such accommodation be encouraged? I believe that insofar as administrative mechanisms can help at all, one that would be at once simple and useful would require the patient to reaffirm periodically his choice of, or choose an alternative to, his medical service practitioner or unit. Where competition among alternatives is impossible, the patient should be obliged to vote confidence or no confidence in his service. Where the latter is the case, a vote of no confidence should bring immediate attention from the outside and corrective action. Where there is competition, choice of alternative services should be weighty enough to represent a significant (though never fatal) blow to the relative success of a practicing unit.

What I have in mind is a mode of providing individual choice with more influence on services than it has had in the past. In the traditional scheme of things, the way the patient can express his satisfaction with his service is poorly designed for the purpose of encouraging the system to meet his needs, for all he can do is of ambiguous meaning and diffuse consequence. The patient either fails to use the available service at all or uses it in an unhappy or resistant frame of mind. The former, nonutilization, cannot be seen clearly as a criticism of the service, for it can reflect lack of need for service as well as lack of confidence or satisfaction. And when the patient uses the service, the frame of mind in which he does is difficult to assess. Thus, utilization is not by itself an adequate means of expressing consumer evaluation. Some choice independent of utilization must be made available to the consumer in order to establish the substance of his satisfaction. Periodic formal assertion of the choice to continue being on the rolls (or of confidence in the service), whether or not services have been utilized extensively, seems to be such an independent method. But that too is not enough as it stands. In the present system, after all, people leave their doctors and drop out of medical care plans, but without much consequence. Lack of consequence seems to be a function of the fact that such decisions to leave are entirely unorganized, so that unless there is extreme and widespread dissatisfaction such scattered individual decisions have little impact. However, if a number of individuals were obliged to choose or vote all at once, their aggregate decision would have considerable impact on the service they have been using.

I suggest that the formal agreement to resubscribe, recontract, or re-enroll, or the formal vote of confidence in services, constitutes an important choice for the patient and that, rather than relying solely on circumstances so extreme as to galvanize him as an individual to complain or to leave the system, the patient should be expected to express formally his satisfaction by periodically reaffirming his desire to be served the way he has been, or by affirming a desire to leave the practice for some other. At the same time, a large segment of the universe of patients should be expected to make this formal choice all at the same time. Thus, even though they choose as individuals rather than as an organized bloc, the very number of individuals choosing all at once would have great consequence for the income or at least reputation of the practice at issue. This may better encourage the providers of care to be closely attentive to the desires of those it is supposed to be serving. Such patient influence, in conjunction with that of profession and administration, would go far toward keeping medical care true to its professed aims.

The Problem of Health Manpower

In making these recommendations I am well aware that I have not touched on many other policy problems, not the least of which lies in the better use of present personnel and the development of new kinds of workers who can move into the vacuum left by the inadequate supply of physician services. Detailed examination of this problem is not possible here, but it is my thesis that a central issue is the dominance of the medical professions—dominance both in the division of labor and in the public eye. Nurses, aides, former medical corpsmen, midwives, social workers, and a variety of other workers could certainly provide many of the services that are now provided primarily by the profession of medicine or that are controlled by it. Present attempts to train more of them should be increased. But in the present scheme of things no effective and widespread program using such workers is possible without the active cooperation of the dominant profession. If the profession does not trust them, or if it resents and fears them, it will not refer patients to them nor will it graciously receive patients referred from them. Given the strategic position of the profession in health services, mere administrative fiat establishing the right of other occupations to supply health services is not enough to assure integrated and coordinated care. Optimal forms of coordination of health services require that physicians be positively interested in working with other personnel. Indeed, without positive encouragement by physicians, I find it hard to believe that most laymen will make willing and comfortable use of other health workers.

The few recommendations I have made are designed to interest the dominant profession in making better use of available health workers. Requiring high technical and humane standards of practice discourages the cutting of medical, psychological, and social corners by physicians attempting to cope with an over-heavy work load. Without the safety valve of corner-cutting, other devices must be used, the most obvious of which lie in passing over much of the load to other workers. Thus, with the establishment of its responsibility to the administrative representatives of the public as well as its responsibility to the individual patient, and with tying rewards to the competent and humane service of both, I believe that the profession might itself undertake partial solution to the problem of manpower now facing the nation by offering other health workers greater responsibility, autonomy, and dignity in a truly collaborative relationship.

All of this, of course, presumes that the medical profession will cooperate with the institution of a new system based on the principles of professional review of the quality of care and of responsiveness to patients' needs. It may not be willing to cooperate, and, as Badgley and Wolfe[8] have shown in one case, its resistance can have serious consequences for the implementation of a new scheme. Should the possibility of professional resistance to the realization of its own ideals be great, then a considerably more modest program of change would seem necessary, change that slowly diminishes the substance of the profession's monopoly over services. The bulk of the everyday medical diagnosis and prescription in primary medical practice, and at least some of the routine forms of surgery, can be performed adequately by a variety of trained nurses, assistants, midwives, corpsmen, and the like. Continued efforts should be made to train and license such practitioners for *independent* practice and to strengthen the position of practitioners outside the medical division of labor, restricting medicine's monopoly to the more esoteric and specialized tasks for which its elaborate education and limited numbers best equip it. The availability to the patient of these new practitioners in the face of the patent inadequacy of available medical services will, no doubt slowly, but in time, come to drain off much of the demand for everyday physician services. Ultimately, this will also reduce the capacity of the profession to resist effectively the institution of a system intended to approach the ideal of competent health service in the interest of all segments of the lay public.

Professional Dominance and Health Care

In this chapter I have recommended that no matter what the concrete insurance, payment, and practice arrangements may be, it is essential that any future system of medical care in the United States be freely available to all irrespective of income and that it provide both technically competent and humanly decent service. I suggested that such care could be encouraged by competition among practitioners or practice units for patients and tempered by the requirement of periodic review of practitioner performance by visiting representatives of the profession. I also recommended that methods be instituted to insure that the response of individual patients to their care has significant impact on the fortunes of those who provide their care. And finally, I suggested that with, or if necessary without, the cooperation of the dominant profession, other occupations to provide health care be developed and strengthened.

The aim of my recommendations is to keep medical care true to the professed ideals of those who dominate it. They have been designed to accommodate to a great variety of concrete economic and organizational schemes in such a way as to minimize the undesirable consequences likely to flow from any particular scheme. Underlying the substance of those recommendations is the conclusion of my extended analysis of medicine as a dominant profession: by their very nature, professions in general and medicine in particular cannot live up to their professed ideals as long as they possess thoroughgoing autonomy to control the terms and content of their work and as long as they are dominant in a division of labor. In essence, I suggested ways by which professional dominance and autonomy could be tempered by administrative accountability, by accountability to the individual patient himself, and by the deliberate encouragement of workers who can compete with the medical practitioner.

It may be argued that the reduction of professional autonomy and dominance would in essence destroy the capacity of professionals to do their indubitably valuable work properly. There is indeed a real danger of such destruction were sheer know-nothingism to prevail. But certainly something must be done to reorganize the rigid and unresponsive modes by which health care is now provided. No matter what their capacities, physicians are not now doing their work properly: reforms are necessary to bring more care to all segments of the population at a reasonable cost and to assure the quality of that care. In the process of formulating and implementing reform the profession is hardly so weak as to be incapable of defending itself. Ultimately, its strongest ally is its own demonstrable knowledge and skill. Its technical achievements in medicine and surgery are such as to create the possibility of a longer and more comfortable (even if not better) life for all men. Those achievements, and the knowledge and skill on which they are based, are worth respect and support. The problem lies in the profession's claim of authority in areas where achievement is by no means so self-evident.

As I have noted earlier in this book, it seems to be in the nature of professionally organized authority to rely on the force and prerogatives of its official status rather than to undertake the wearisome effort of persuading and demonstrating. Organized medicine, both in the United States and elsewhere, is a prime example of such a tendency, a tendency that, in conjunction with its dominance over jurisdictional issues in health affairs, has brought us to the present state of crisis in health services. It asserts its control over the performance of medical work at the same time its practitioners are too few to perform the work. It refuses to allow members of other occupations to perform such work except in a position of subordination from which they can gain little satisfaction. It insists on its jurisdiction over everything related to that vague word "health," including that vast, undifferentiated problem called "mental illness" for which neither medicine nor any other discipline has demonstrated any consistently effective therapeutic solution.[9] When its powers outstrip its capacity to perform satisfactorily, the claims on which they rest cannot fail to seem hypocritical.

The present system of organizing health care relies too

much on the dominance of medical authority in a context of diffuse responsibility and accountability. Only reorganization of the terms and mechanisms of the system can provide an environment in which the profession can be more honest and its service better. Such a reorganized system consists of an administrative framework that maintains the legitimate prerogatives of the professional worker while insisting on his essential obligation to regulate himself in the service of the public. And not least of all, it establishes the essential right, indeed obligation, of the patient to serve as an active participant in the process of shaping the services that are supposed to exist for his benefit.

NOTES

1. For an attempt to review the available American material, see Eliot Freidson, "The Organization of Medical Practice," in Howard Freeman et al., eds., *Handbook of Medical Sociology* (Englewood Cliffs, N. J.: Prentice-Hall, 1970), rev. ed., and its bibliography.
2. See the very extensive argument in Eliot Freidson, *Profession of Medicine: A Study of the Sociology of Applied Knowledge* (New York: Dodd-Mead, 1970). See also the important work on a variety of professions in Corinne Lathrop Gilb, *Hidden Hierarchies: The Professions and Government* (New York: Harper & Row, 1966).
3. See, for example, "Utilization Review and Control Activities in Blue Cross Plans," *Blue Cross Reports*, 4 (January–March 1966), 1–12.
4. For a recent brief review of other countries, see Max Seham, "An American Doctor Looks at Eleven Foreign Health Systems," *Social Science and Medicine*, 3 (1969), 65–81. See also J. Hogarth, *The Payment of the Physician, Some European Comparisons* (New York: Pergamon, 1963).
5. See, for example, the discussion of the literature in Peter M. Blau and W. Richard Scott, *Formal Organizations* (San Francisco, Calif.: Chandler, 1962).

6. Group practice on any significant scale has not expanded rapidly in the United States or elsewhere, most physicians apparently preferring the independence they can feel in solo or small partnership practice. See the Dutch survey, P. M. Verbeek-Heida, "General Practitioners' Attitudes toward Group Practice in the Netherlands," *Social Science and Medicine*, 3 (1969), 249–258.
7. In this context I may cite the temperate and sensible comments on planning in David Mechanic, "Some Notes on the Future of General Medical Practice in the United States," *Inquiry*, 6 (1969), 22–25.
8. Robin F. Badgley and Samuel Wolfe, *Doctors' Strike, Medical Care and Conflict in Saskatchewan* (New York: Atherton Press, 1967).
9. An extremely good evaluation of the field of mental health and its policy problems has recently been made in David Mechanic, *Mental Health and Social Policy* (Englewood Cliffs, N. J.: Prentice-Hall, 1969). Especially relevant for my discussion are his comments on the mental health division of labor and his contrast between the medical and the educational models for managing the mental patient.

Index

Administrative organization, of medical care, 222–225
Ambulatory medical care, organizing, 187–208
Ambulatory services, barriers to free choice of, 192–196
American Sociological Association, Medical Sociology Section, 45
Associations, professional, 82, 83
Authority
  expert, 108
  official, 108
  professional
    institutional impurities in, 115–118
    levels of, 121–123
    problem of, structural solution to, 105–126
  scientific, 123–125
Autonomy, organized, profession as, 133–135

Barriers to a sociology of medicine, 50–53
Becker, Howard S., 86
Belknap, Ivan, 171, 174
Blau, Peter, 130
Boycott, 94, 95, 99–100
Bucher, Rue, 16
Bureaucracy
  advisory, 25
  professionalism and, 23–25, 90, 129–133
  rational-legal, Weber's analysis of, 23–24, 108–109, 130

Carlin, Jerome, 133
Carr-Sanders, A. M., 94, 97
Cartwright, Ann, 180
Caudill, William, 173
Client-dependent practice, 91, 92
Client services, bias in, 145–151
Clients
  health organization and, 137–141
  role in medical services, 225–231
  see also Patients
Clinic organization, traditional, 196–199
Coleman, James, 19, 89
Colleague-dependent practice, 91–93
Colleague networks, 89, 100–101
Columbia University, medical education study, 84
Common-sense individualism, 59–60, 64, 65, 67
Community
  health and the, 30–31
  hospital organization as a, 27–29
Competition, medical care, 220–222
Consultant role, 14–15
Consultation, profession of, 106–108
Coser, Rose L., 27–28, 178
Cultural differences, between physician and patients, 110–113

Cumming, Elaine, 30
Cumming, John, 30

Davis, Fred, 142
Depersonalization of patients, 169–172
Disease
  concept of, 3–5
  as ideology, 5–8
  prevention of, 31
Division of labor, *see* Labor, division of
Doctor-patient relationship, 15
  professional authority and, 105–126
Doctors, *see* Physicians
Dominance, professional
  division of labor and, 135–137
  health care and, 233–236
  health services and, 127–164
  reorganization of medical care and, 209–237

Eaton, Joseph W., 9, 30
Education, medical, 16–18, 84–87
Educational differences, between physician and patients, 110–113
Environment, survival and, 61–62
Evans, J. W., 19
Evolution, theory of, 61, 62

Financing, medical care, 216–220
Free choice
  of ambulatory services, barriers to, 192–196
  significance of, 120–121
Freeman, Howard, 9
Freidson, Eliot, 19, 94
Freud, Sigmund, 6

Georgopoulos, Basil S., 175, 176
Goals, medical service, 212–215
Goffman, Erving, 28–29, 169
Goss, Mary E. W., 24–25, 130
Gouldner, Alvin W., 130
Group practice, 199–206

Hall, Oswald, 19, 89
Healing role, 15
Health, community and, 30–31
Health care, professional dominance and, 233–236
Health organization, clients and, 137–141
Health services
  organization of, 1–2
  professional dominance and, 127–164
Hippias, 142
Hospital care
  limiting conditions of, 177–179
  organizing, 167–186
    issues in, 181–185
Hospitals
  depersonalization of patients, 169–172
  organization of, as a community, 27–29
  position of medicine in, 174–176
  sociology of, 22–23, 28
  utopian, 172–174
Hughes, Everett Cherrington, 105, 107, 109, 115, 122, 123

Ideology, disease as, 5–8
Illness
  responses to
    organization of, 11–15
    social class influences on, 10–11
    social elements in distribution and etiology of, 8–9
Individualism, common-sense, 59–60, 64, 65, 67
Information
  professional control of, 141–143
  withholding, from patients, 139–143
Institutions, total, 28

James IV (Scotland), 114

Kansas, University of, 85, 86
Kobler, Arthur L., 174, 175

Labor, division of
  autonomy in, 135–137

professional dominance in, 135–137
Lasswell, Harold D., 172–173
Lefton, Mark, 27
Levine, Sol, 30
Licensing, 83, 134
Lieberson, Stanley, 191

Mann, Floyd C., 175, 176
Manpower, health, problem of, 231–233
Marx, Karl, 25
Medical care
  administrative organization of, 222–225
  ambulatory, organizing, 187–208
  competition in, 220–222
  financing, 216–220
  organizing, problems of, 165–237
  reorganization of
    principles for, 215–216
    professional dominance and, 209–237
  settings of, 31–32
  social structure and, 69–73
  sociological approach to, 39–77
  structural approach to, 59–77
  structure, position of medical profession in, 79–164
  working toward a sociology of, 57–58
Medical policy, social structure and, 66–69
Medical practice, 18–20
  bureaucratic, 90–91
  client-dependent, 91, 92
  colleague-dependent, 91–93
  designing, 74–76
  group, 199–206
  institutionalization of, outcomes of, 118–120
  milieu of, 20
  organization of, 70–74
  professional regulation of, 93–96
  solo, 88–89, 189–192
  types of, 87–93
    analytical, 91–93
    empirical, 87–91
Medical profession
  as an element of social structure, 76–77
  informal organization of the, 99–102
  overview of, 81–104
  position of, in medical care structure, 79–164
  regulation of, 93–96
  values and the, 96–99
Medical schools, 16–18, 84–87
Medical services
  client's role in, 225–231
  goals of, 212–215
Medical sociology
  barriers to, 50–53
  issues in, 1–37
  present state of, 41–58
  tasks of, 53–57, 102–103
  underdevelopment of, 45–50
Medical training, *see* Education, medical; Schools, medical
Medicine
  professionals in, 15–22
  sociology of, differentiated from sociology in, 41–42, 44
  state and, 83–84
  See also Medical sociology
Mental disorder, medical orientation to, 5–6

Newton, Isaac, 5
Nonprofessional workers
  alienation of, 143–145
  motivation of, 25–27
  professional dominance over, 143–145
Nurses, role of, 20–22, 26–27
Nursing, profession of, 20–22

Parsons, Talcott
  on authority, 131, 158
  consultant role described by, 14–15
  on disease, 4
  on professional regulation, 97
  on professional values, 96, 97
  sick role described by, 12–13

Parsons, Talcott (*continued*)
  on Weber's analysis of rational-legal bureaucracy, 23–24, 108–109, 130
Pasteur, Louis, 5
Patients
  depersonalization of, 169–172
  "free choice" and, 120–121, 192–196
  see also Clients
Physicians
  cultural and educational differences between patients and, 110–113
  licensing of, 83, 134
  prestige, professional, 113–115
  professional role of, 15–20
  see also Doctor-patient relationship
Prestige, professional, 113–115
Profession, *see* Medical profession
Professionalism, 21–22
  bureaucracy and, 23–25, 90, 129–133
  limitations on, 158–161
  as organized autonomy, 133–135
  role of, 151–156
  values and, 96–99, 152–154

Regulation, professional, 93–96
Rhea, Buford, 94
Roth, Julius A., 47
Rubenstein, Robert, 172–173

Schizophrenia, 9
Schools
  medical, 16–18, 84–87
  nursing, 21
Schwartz, Morris S., 171
Science, 107–108, 109
Seeman, M., 19, 27
Sick role, 12–14, 15
Simmons, Ozzie, 9
Smigel, Erwin O., 130
Smith, Harvey L., 24
Social class, influences on responses to illness, 10–11
Social elements in distribution and etiology of illness, 8–9
Social epidemiology, 46
Social structure
  medical care and, 69–73
  medical policy and, 66–69
  profession as an element of, 76–77
Sociology
  of hospitals, 22–23, 28
  of medicine, differentiated from sociology in medicine, 41–42, 44
  see also Medical sociology
Solo practice, 88–89
  organization of, 189–192
Specialists, 71–72
  choice of career by, 87
  client-dependent, 92
  colleague-dependent, 92
Stanton, Alfred H., 171
State, medicine and the, 83–84
Status differences, between physician and patients, 113–115
Steinle, John G., 174
Stotland, Ezra, 174, 175
Straus, Robert, 41
Strauss, Anselm, 16, 171
Stress, 5
Survival, environment and, 61–62
Syndicalism, professional, 76

Tasks, of medical sociology, 53–57, 102–103
Thompson, Victor, 130
Thorner, I., 20
Total institutions, 28
Training, medical, *see* Education, medical; Schools, medical

Underdevelopment of medical sociology, 45–50

Values, professional, 96–99, 152–154

Weber, Max, 23, 25, 108, 130
Weil, R. J., 9, 30
White, Paul E., 30
Wilson, P. A., 94, 97
Workers, nonprofessional, *see* Nonprofessional workers